PRAISE FOR PURE TEENS

Pure Teens: Free to Love, by Dr. John Thorington, is an outstanding resource for Christian teens and their parents. What makes this book unique is the way it is organized into 28 daily segments that invite shared reading and reflection by teens and their parents. In today's world, Christian youth need their parents' loving presence and support more than ever. Together, Christian families can explore the challenges faced by every family as children develop sexually, including sexual temptation, masturbation and following God's plan for the healthy expression of our sexuality. *Pure Teens: Free to Love* should be in every home where children are growing into sexual responsibility and maturity.

Rev. David Rennard, LCSW, CSAT-S

Pure Teens: Free to Love, by Dr. John Thorington, is a bold new book with practical and accurate information on the effects of sexuality on the mind and spirit of the teen. This is a great resource for any parent looking for a biblical resource to help their teen find hope and healing from sexual temptation, lust, and experimentation. I would also recommend this book to any adult who struggles with sexual purity.

Rev. George Stahnke, founder of Renewal Ministries of Colorado Springs

Dr. Thorington tackles the sensitive and delicate topics of masturbation and lust in a very teen-understandable and balanced way: spiritually and scientifically, laying out a clear end goal and validating the struggle to get there. *Pure Teens: Free to Love* encourages humility, commitment, faith which are all to be covered with God's grace for the journey.

Timothy Sanford, MA. Author of *Forgive for Real, INSIDE: Understanding How Reactive Attachment Disorder Thinks and Feels* and *Losing Control and Liking It: Setting Your Teen and Yourself Free.*

John Thorington's new book *Pure Teens: Free to Love* is phenomenal. As a parent of a teenage boy, this is the first book I have been able to find that speaks so very directly on a topic that Christians rarely talk about. He not only clearly gives the big picture of God's plan for healthy sexuality, but also breaks it down and is able to provide scientific evidence on the harmful effects of pornography on the brain. John's book provides hope and freedom for teens that feel that they are trapped in a downward cycle. It also equips parents with tools on how to engage in dialogue on what is sometimes an extremely uncomfortable topic.

The discussion starters are an excellent way to think through questions teens and parents don't normally ask themselves. I think this book is a must read for every parent that wants to help their child have a healthy view of sexuality, that honors God and builds a healthy foundation for a future marriage.

Sayeh Sparr, MSW

Pure Teens: Free to Love is a great resource to help teenagers begin conversations around masturbation, with daily readings and questions to spark discussion. This book helps teens evaluate and talk through their own attitudes and behaviors to determine what they may want to change. Then, Dr. Thorington provides empathy for the common teen struggle with masturbation while providing concrete steps to help them overcome it.

John Fort, Director of Training, Be Broken Ministries

PURE TEENS
FREE TO LOVE

DR. JOHN THORINGTON

WESTBOW
PRESS®
A DIVISION OF THOMAS NELSON
& ZONDERVAN

WestBow Press books may be ordered through booksellers or by contacting:

WestBow Press
A Division of Thomas Nelson & Zondervan
1663 Liberty Drive
Bloomington, IN 47403
www.westbowpress.com
1 (866) 928-1240

ISBN: 978-1-9736-7714-7 (sc)
ISBN: 978-1-9736-7716-1 (hc)
ISBN: 978-1-9736-7715-4 (e)

Library of Congress Control Number: 2019915931

Print information available on the last page.

WestBow Press rev. date: 10/28/2019

INTRODUCTION

In today's sex-saturated culture, you need a plan of action for living purely. I published *Pure Teens: Honoring God, Relationships, and Sex* back in 2016 to help teens in this battle for their spiritual identity and destiny.

Pure Teens: Free to Love is, in many ways, a companion to that book, though it will surely benefit teens who haven't read the first book. The book addresses these four topics below one week at a time in the daily readings:

1. How to View Masturbation and Lust
2. What the Scripture Says about Lust
3. Winning Strategies for the Battle
4. God's Design for Sacred Sex

Although sexual thoughts and feelings are healthy, it's a great challenge to acquire a godly mind-set in today's world. Your sexuality is a central part of who you are as a human being, and how you use your God-given gift will determine your life to a remarkable degree.

As a person who served in pastoral ministry for thirty years, I know of no greater failure in the church than not presenting a positive and God-honoring perspective about sexuality. God is calling your generation to know who you are and what you believe as His people.

In this book, you will find valuable information and practical suggestions about how to live lust-free. There are twenty-eight daily readings, and you can choose your own pace. You may want to spend more time than a day reflecting on some of the specific readings.

More importantly, you will be guided through some discussions of great magnitude. Each of the weeks in *Pure Teens: Free to Love* will help you to figure out God's road map for you in making decisions about your sexual integrity.

The goal is to promote healthy discussion between teens and their parents. For too long, the approach of most parents has been a "don't ask, don't tell" policy. This has been the dominant pattern within the church too. Sadly, the world has taken over the role of educating young people about relationships and sexuality. It is time that we reclaimed this lost territory based on God's abiding Word.

The material in the Discussion Starters at the end of each daily reading is intended to bring you to a closer relationship with the God who deeply loves you. It is also a tool to help facilitate healthy relationship building and communication between teens and their parents.

The most effective use of this book is for both the parent and the teen to read the daily material and go through the questions together. Some will read the daily material and then talk. Some parents will literally read the daily content out loud with their teens before discussing it. The material provides a basis for what is most important—the conversation between parents and teens. The goal is for healthy dialogue in a safe, caring environment where the parent doesn't lecture. Instead, the goal is to have a conversation about this life-changing subject.

Some churches will likely use this resource as a curriculum. That is exciting too. Again, it is hoped that parents will be involved in the dialogue and teaching.

I congratulate you for opening this book and taking that first step toward living a lust-free life. You are about to learn how to navigate some of the big stuff of life—lust, fantasy, masturbation, and premarital sex. In the pages that follow, you will learn to view sexuality within the overall biblical narrative and the invitation to follow Jesus!

It is my prayer that you will come to know the God who is wildly in love with you. He couldn't possibly love you more—His is a perfect, awe-inspiring, and completely satisfying love! Further, as Paul says, "For this reason I kneel before the Father.... I pray that out of his glorious riches he may strengthen you with power through his Spirit in your inner being" (Eph. 3:14, 16).

CONTENTS

WEEK THREE
STRATEGIES FOR ALL WHO STRUGGLE

WEEK FOUR
GOD'S DESIGN FOR SEX

WEEK ONE
HOW BIG A DEAL ARE LUST AND MASTURBATION?

DAY 1
WHO MASTURBATES AND WHY?

Masturbation is, in many ways, a taboo topic. It isn't something that we readily talk about in our families and churches. Yet masturbation is prevalent. Just how frequent does masturbation happen among teens?

Dr. Cynthia Robbins serves in the pediatrics department at Indiana University, and she led the first national study of masturbation among teens. The research involved more than eight hundred American teens ranging in age from fourteen to seventeen and discovered the following results:

- Across fourteen- to seventeen-year-olds, 74 percent of the boys and 48 percent of the girls reported masturbating.
- Among males, masturbation increased with age: just 63 percent of the younger boys reported masturbating at least once, but the figure rose to 80 percent among seventeen-year-olds.
- In females, the percentage also rose with age, from 43 percent for fourteen-year-olds to 58 percent for seventeen-year-olds. [1]

The research indicates a high occurrence of masturbation among teens. So who masturbates? Let's start by saying that, from a personal development point of view, almost everybody at one time in life has masturbated. And why? Several reasons can be cited:

- It is a normal part of a child's exploration of his or her body.
- Teens learn how their bodies can produce pleasure.
- Some use masturbation to lower stress and help themselves relax.
- Males and females engage in masturbation as a form of safe sex—solo sex.

We gain some clarification by viewing life in two developmental stages: self-discovery and young adulthood. The first stage is self-discovery during ages thirteen to seventeen. Here a kid's body goes through changes during puberty. There are both physical and psychological changes during this stage. For example, teens become sexually aware and more interested in the opposite sex. Masturbation in the self-discovery stage is typically driven by curiosity, and parents are encouraged to communicate in a nonshaming way.

Masturbation is far more prevalent in the young adult stage, with approximate ages eighteen to twenty-four. The natural drive for sex becomes stronger in this stage of development. At this stage, masturbation is nearly universal for guys and quite common for girls. There is no need for a person to be burdened with self-condemnation. Most guys and girls work through this stage and maintain their relationship with God. The problem arises when lust and masturbation become deeply rooted.

For the sake of clarity, let's use the following definition of *masturbation*. *Merriam-Webster's Medical Dictionary* states that it is

> Erotic stimulation of one's own genital organs commonly resulting in orgasm and achieved by manual or other bodily contact exclusive of

sexual intercourse, by instrumental manipulation, occasionally by sexual fantasies.[2]

Most churches don't talk about sexual things, such as masturbation, lust, or pornography. Some of the churches that do speak on these matters do so from a sex-negative perspective. They make or imply nonsensical comments such as, "Sex is bad, so save it for the one you love." That is *not* a biblical view in any way!

Christian teens mainly struggle without the support of the church or parents. Natural curiosity may get the better of them as their bodies are going through raging hormonal and physical changes. It can be awkward to share one's thoughts and feelings with a parent or youth pastor. Where do teens turn for help?

No wonder most teens are searching the internet for answers to avoid the embarrassment. Looking online for information about sex is risky and can have harmful consequences as the cyberworld extensively promotes a wide-open path to the pursuit of self-gratification. A balanced and healthy perspective on masturbation is often lacking.

Teens need the support of their parents and the church regarding sexual matters. Howard Henricks stated, "We should not be ashamed to talk about what God wasn't ashamed to create."[3] His comment is a challenge to the church and parents to address the holy nature of sex. God created sex, and He has an excellent design for all His children.

It is the responsibility of first parents and then the church to offer guidance to teens on masturbation and other sexual matters. It doesn't work to have a policy of "Don't ask, don't tell" or "just say no." Teens need help to understand what's happening to their bodies as a part of God's great and perfect design.

This book will provide biblical and scientific information about sex, masturbation, and porn. Hopefully, the questions at the end of each day will help you to acquire a biblical mind-set. Just maybe, it will help encourage some healthy conversation between you and your parents.

DISCUSSION STARTERS

1. What does the research tell us about the prevalence of masturbation?
2. Do you see any danger in using only the internet for sex education?
3. Is there some advantage of looking at this topic from a developmental stage perspective involving self-discovery and young adulthood?
4. Do you agree with Howard Hendrix that God doesn't want us to look at sexuality through the lens of shame?

DAY 2
OPPOSING VIEWPOINTS

Many people have a hard time saying "the m word": *masturbation.* The word usually raises a mixed response from people. It is often softly spoken, laughed about, or expressed with shame. Masturbation is a normal behavior among teens.

Most people discover masturbation in adolescence. There are two unhealthy perspectives that we want to avoid. The first view is characterized by embarrassment and shame. It is communicated in false statements such as the following:

- "Masturbation is harmful to your health."
- "You'll grow lots of hair or warts on your palms."
- "Other people will know by simply looking at you."
- "Masturbation is always a sin."
- "Masturbation will cause you to lose your eyesight."
- "Masturbation is not natural."

It is honest to say that the traditional scare tactics regarding masturbation lack credibility. It would be better for us to reflect on this issue from a biblical perspective.

Let's be compassionate and honest in our discussion on this very personal matter. The Bible states,

> Therefore, there is now no condemnation for those
> who are in Christ Jesus, because through Christ
> Jesus the law of the Spirit who gives life has set you
> free from the law of sin and death. (Rom. 8:1–2)

There won't be any guilt imposed on you if you struggle with masturbation. Your relationship with God is not determined by the degree of success or failure in measuring up to His moral standard. That's good news for all of us!

Now, is there a character example to which God calls us? Yes, God calls us to grow in character like His Son Jesus. Scripture encourages us to "flee from sexual immorality" (1 Cor. 6:18). Jesus boldly warned against staring at a woman, or any person for that matter, with lust in our hearts (Matt. 5:28). However, we must not confuse our salvation as being based upon the victory over sin by our efforts and achievements. The triumph is and always will be the result of God's grace through Christ for humble, repentant sinners. "If we confess our sins, he is faithful and just and will forgive us our sins and purify us from all unrighteousness" (1 John 1:9).

Here is a compelling biblical story that will give you some idea of God's grace. Jesus in His public ministry was ever so tender toward struggling sinners, even as He convicted their hypocritical accusers. There was a group of Pharisees and religious leaders who brought a woman caught in the act of adultery. They sought to trap Jesus, so they asked Him what to do with her. According to the law of Moses, it was an option to stone her to death. Jesus replied, "Let any one of you who is without sin be the first to throw a stone at her" (John 8:7b). Jesus expresses great love and mercy!

Like Jesus, we want to discuss sexual issues with both compassion and truth. Jesus didn't judge this woman when she was vulnerable and exposed to public humiliation. Her very life was at stake. Jesus protected her and rescued her—literally saved her life that day! Yes, we want to create a caring environment where all who have sexual struggles can feel safe and find help.

The other misleading perspective is one that supports masturbation with no reservations. The world's attitude is akin to the idea, "If it feels good, do it." Proponents of this distorted opinion assert that masturbation is a normal and healthy sexual activity for men and women. According to this view, it is pleasurable, acceptable, and safe with no exceptions.

This unqualified view is naive at best and harmful at worst. While masturbation is a natural behavior, it can be a real problem. Most of us would agree that masturbation is problematic and risky when it

- happens in public,
- results in self-injury,
- interferes with daily life and activities,
- shapes sexual interests in harmful ways,
- conflicts with faith-based principles,
- develops into an addiction, or
- combines with pornographic images.

Why discuss this subject? Is masturbation really a big deal? Several years ago, highly respected Dr. James Dobson with Focus on the Family wrote,

> It is my opinion that masturbation is not much of an issue with God. It is a normal part of adolescence, which involves no one else. It does not cause disease, it does not produce babies, and Jesus did not mention it in the Bible. I'm not telling you to masturbate, and I hope you don't feel the need for it. The best thing I can do is suggest that you talk to God personally about this matter and decide what He wants you to do.[4]

Dr. Dobson is a highly esteemed Christian leader throughout the world. His perspective on masturbation was influenced by his dad, who was trying to spare him of the legalism in his church upbringing. We appreciate his father's intention of saving his son from experiencing unhealthy shame. However, strictly speaking, it is theologically incorrect to broadly say that "masturbation is not much of an issue with God." God cares deeply about every part of our lives—especially when it comes to the matter of sexual expression!

Is masturbation a big deal or not? The short answer is, in some ways it is and some ways it is not. It is something that impacts you and most teens. It would help if you decided what is healthy for you in the long run. What is God's will for you?

God provided the precious gift of sexuality to be protected and enjoyed. Paul states, "Therefore, I urge you, brothers and sisters, in view of God's mercy, to offer your bodies as a living sacrifice, holy and pleasing to God—this is your true and proper worship" (Rom. 12:1).

Some Christians make too big a deal and miss the more significant issues of the heart. Men and women can obsess over how many times they have masturbated. God wants you to be far more concerned about the condition of your heart. God is passionately longing for you to give your heart completely to Him (see Deut. 6:5).

DISCUSSION STARTERS

1. Do you think that masturbation is all right without any reservations?
2. Are their times when masturbation can be a problem?
3. What difference does it make to believe that your body belongs to the Lord (Rom. 12:1)?
4. Do you understand and agree with the idea that God cares mostly about giving your heart to Him?

DAY 3

WHEN IS MASTURBATION HARMFUL?

The following comments are especially applicable if you have been viewing pornography accompanied by masturbation. The combination of pornography and masturbation changes the chemistry in your brain.

For most teens struggling with out-of-control behavior, masturbation is a deep-rooted habit. There are often hundreds of hours with repeating self-stimulation and sexual fantasy states connected to this robust conditioning process. This behavior can lead to a neurochemical imbalance. The continuation of masturbation can make it very difficult to change the lustful thought patterns.

In many cases, stopping masturbation is necessary for preventing the compulsive use of pornography. If you have been masturbating for two or three years, this process will take time and support. Is it that important?

A significant number of teens have reported that continuing to masturbate has undermined their sexual integrity. Masturbation helped to drive their fantasies and often served as a stimulus to other types of acting out. You are encouraged to carefully consider this fact in making your decision about the practice of masturbation.

Whether your masturbation is healthy or harmful depends on numerous factors. A key consideration is the frequency of the behavior. If you are asking "How many times a day can I masturbate?" the question itself indicates a habitual pattern. You are encouraged to examine what you are doing and its impact. You may decide that masturbation is harmful to your spiritual journey.

More specifically, whether the masturbation is harmful or healthy depends to a large extent on what you are thinking about or viewing when you do it. If you are masturbating with porn images or fantasies in your mind, then it is an issue. This pattern usually leads to isolated, self-centered, and unrealistic sexual experiences.

The words of Jesus are very appropriate to this discussion. He said, "But I tell you that anyone who looks at a woman lustfully has already committed adultery with her in his heart" (Matt. 5:28). Jesus cares deeply about your heart and that you learn to walk the path of love. He said, "By this everyone will know that you are my disciples, if you love one another" (John 13:35). Love and lust cannot coexist in your heart. Lust will always damage or destroy love.

You may be among the many teens whose acting out is primarily masturbation and viewing pornography. Several researchers have observed that those who struggle the most with compulsive behavior are those who act out with "only" masturbation and watching pornography. Masturbation fueled by fantasy can be very addictive and hard to stop for those obsessed with it.

You will need to decide whether to stop masturbation. The information provided in this book can help you make a wise choice. The resources are intended to help you find a sexual expression that is psychologically healthy, socially responsible, intimacy enhancing, and spiritually fulfilling.

How you answer the questions below may help in making your decision about masturbation. You alone can make this decision. If it is going to be part of your life, you are encouraged to discuss this with your parents or a therapist to determine whether it is wise or not. If you choose not to masturbate, identify the boundaries you want to establish to remove this habit from your life.

The directions for this questionnaire are simple. There is a series of questions, and you are asked to check either yes or no for each one. Read the statements and indicate your response.

QUESTIONNAIRE:

		Yes	No
1.	Am I trying to medicate or numb my feelings?	___	___
2.	Will I feel ashamed afterward?	___	___
3.	Am I relying on fantasy or porn to masturbate?	___	___
4.	Am I doing this to release stress?	___	___
5.	When I masturbate, do I go on a binge?	___	___
6.	Am I becoming more "me-centered"?	___	___
7.	Am I breaking a boundary necessary for my integrity?	___	___
8.	Am I more out of touch with my feelings?	___	___
9.	Am I dishonoring God as I masturbate?	___	___
10.	Am I creating a problem for my future marriage?	___	___

If you answered yes to any of the above questions, you are encouraged to discuss your responses with your parents or a therapist. We know this may not be an honest discussion without some discomfort, but it is an important one.

What will be your decision about masturbation? Did the questions help you to process essential factors in your decision making? What do you think God is saying to you about this issue?

DISCUSSION STARTERS

1. Do you understand how the combination of pornography and masturbation is complicated to stop from a neurochemical perspective?
2. Did you answer yes to any of the ten questions? If so, will you discuss those statements with your parents or a therapist?
3. Can you explain the significance of Jesus' words in Matthew 5:28? (Go back and read the text.)
4. What will be your understanding and practice regarding masturbation?

DAY 4
SEX AND THE BRAIN

You will need at least a simple understanding of the brain to live a pure life. Teens now have the facts to steer them away from making life-altering mistakes and lead them toward reaching their full potential.

Until recently, there wasn't much evidence or research to reach reliable conclusions. That has changed with lots of new and exciting studies. One helpful resource is the book *The Drug of the New Millennium: The Science of How Internet Pornography Radically Alters the Human Brain and Body* (2001) by Mark B. Kasselman. If you want to learn more about sex and the brain, you are encouraged to read this book.

We have known for many years that sex was more than a physical experience. However, there was no real way of knowing what was happening in the brain when people were engrossed in love, passion, lust, sexual feelings, or other emotions. Now we know considerably more due to recent studies and neuroscience.

Could it be that the apostle Paul understood the drug-like effect of pornography and masturbation? He said, "Flee from sexual immorality. All other sins a person commits are outside the body, but whoever sins sexually, sins against their own body" (1 Cor. 6:18). Some have suggested this refers to sexually transmitted diseases (STDs), including HIV/AIDS. Undoubtedly, sexual behaviors outside the will of God can result in disease and even death.

There is something else intended for us to understand in this scripture. What we are talking about is the field of neuroscience and the many advances of the past several years. You will see that there is significant scientific support for the Bible's teaching on the brain and sex. Let's look and better understand what 1 Corinthians 6:18 says about the mind.

We now know that "sex produces powerful, even lifelong, changes in our brains that direct and influence our future to a surprising degree."[5] This is a good reason for learning about the connection between sex and our brains.

Today, thanks to breakthroughs in neuroscience, scientists have been able to view the activity of the brain as it functions. Researchers have been able to unlock a whole new world of data. Here are five things you should know about pornography and the brain:

1. Pornography releases life-changing chemicals that can hook you. At the time of a sexual release, the brain receives a rush of chemicals. The most critical chemical in the brain concerning reward is dopamine (the feel-good chemical). It also influences your behavior, cognition, and motivation. Sex is one of the most potent producers of the dopamine reward. Teens are especially vulnerable to viewing pornography and getting hooked because it creates a high feeling.

2. Sexual images get imprinted in the DNA of your brain. We know from neuroscience that sexual imprinting takes place when you look at pornography. The unfortunate reality is that when you look at porn and act it out (say, by masturbating), this has hormonal and neurological consequences. In short, you are designed to bond with the object to which you give your focus and attention. In God's design, this would be your spouse, but for many teens, it is an image on the screen.

3.   The stimulation of pornography hurts relational and sexual satisfaction. We know from the research that dopamine surges as a person views different sorts of pornography. The prospect for a satisfying and lasting relationship lessens with exposure to erotic images that trigger more dopamine than a long-term partner. Thus, what God intended to be the ultimate pleasure is replaced by porn images and fantasy. Can you see what Paul was talking about in 1 Corinthians 6:18?

4.   Pornography takes you where you don't want to go. Why do guys and girls seek out a variety of new sexual images rather than being satisfied with the same ones? Neuroscience helps us to understand what has been called the *Coolidge effect*. It is a neurological effect (again, the brain is changed) where the teen has renewed sexual interest when introduced to new partners. The sad impact of this is that teens eventually find themselves looking at and getting aroused by very degrading and dehumanizing images.

5.   Pornography is very harmful to your brain's development and function. What makes porn unique and especially dangerous for teens? Gary Wilson identifies a number of factors: (1) internet porn delivers extreme novelty; (2) there is almost an endless supply of porn to consume, unlike food and drugs; (3) with internet porn, one can increase consumption both with more novel "partners" and by viewing new and unusual types; and (4) the age at which teens begin viewing porn leaves a lasting imprint. A teen's brain is at its height of dopamine production and neuroplasticity, making it especially vulnerable to addiction and rewiring. [6]

What does the word *neuroplasticity* mean? It doesn't mean our brains are made of plastic, of course! It means that viewing pornography, sexting, and fantasizing about sexual situations can lead to long-lasting changes in the mind that impact memory and learning. When you sin sexually, this is stamped on the brain.

Many teens have discovered that the images are impossible to forget. This is what neuroplasticity is about—it describes any change in final neural activity or behavioral response. Pornography has a significant influence on the brain. The impact, whether for good or bad, depends on what we give our focus and attention. Your choices have durable power to determine your brain development and function.

Nancy Andreasen put it this way: "We can change who and what we do by what we see, hear, say, and do. It is important to choose the activities for our brains to be well trained.... We make choices that change our brains and ultimately change who we are."[7]

DISCUSSION STARTERS

1. What do you think Paul meant when he said, "Flee from sexual immorality. All other sins a man commits are outside of his body, but he who sins sexually sins against his own body" (1 Cor. 6:18)?
2. Can you put into your own words the five things from research that you can learn about pornography and the brain?
3. What is your understanding of neuroplasticity and its importance to your sexuality?
4. How do lust and fantasy change who you are? Your future?

DAY 5
THE BIGGER PICTURE

Most of us agree that the universal desire of humans is to love and be loved. When we feel securely loved by another and free to express our love, this is to be wholly alive. Irenaeus (AD 130–202) was the bishop of Lugdunum in Gaul (modern Lyons, France). He was a strong proponent for biblical truth, and he stated triumphantly, "The glory of God is a human fully alive."[8]

Jesus indeed emphasized this when He said God's great desire for us is to "love the Lord our God with all our heart, soul, mind, and strength" (Mark 12:30). The Bible repeatedly illustrates God's great, passionate, and relentless attraction to us. John wants us to be assured of His love so much so that he writes, "There is no fear in love. But perfect love drives out fear because fear has to do with punishment. The one who fears is not made perfect in love" (1 John 4:18).

Many today are making a very costly exchange in getting involved with sexual sin. We substitute an intimate and life-giving relationship with God for a few seconds of self-gratification.

Porn and masturbation may bring momentary pleasure. But in the end, they leave you empty with feelings of despair and shame. Lust, by its very nature, cannot satisfy. C. S. Lewis described lustful desire with a warning: "The danger is that of coming to love the prison."[9] God created us to be free to love and be loved.

You may have seen the story of Eric Liddell, the Olympic

runner, highlighted in the Oscar-winning movie *Chariots of Fire*. He once made this comment: "When I run, I feel God's pleasure."[10] He made this comment affirming his deep personal desire to please God. In fact, Liddell was more driven by his faith than any desire to win an Olympic gold medal.

His faith prompted him to believe that, since Abba Father gave him this unique ability to run, God took genuine pleasure in watching him use that gift. He felt in his heart that God was delighted whenever he ran and gave it his best effort. There was a vital connection in Liddell's mind between pleasing God and the remarkable energy he felt whenever he ran.

Seen from Liddell's faith-perspective, we understand that the source of his motivation and pleasure in running was his desire to please God. In fact, he refused to run a qualifying heat on a Sunday because he believed in the observance of the Sabbath. While he gave up a medal opportunity, he did go on to win the four-hundred-meter dash on a different day.

The ultimate mark of his life happened a bit later. He left for China a year after the Olympics to serve as a missionary in China. Unfortunately, the Japanese occupied China, and he became interned in a prisoner-of-war camp during WWII. He was a constant source of encouragement to many, establishing a school and sporting activities for the children who were also imprisoned. Sadly, his life ended due to a brain tumor a few months before the Allied troops arrived in China. Another fellow missionary said that Liddell's last words were "It's complete surrender,"[11] referring to his relationship with God.

Liddell was enthused by an awareness that God loved him and gifted him to serve others. He was delighted to use his gifts in honor of God. His life reflected the words of the psalmist, who put it this way:

> I keep my eyes always on the LORD.
> With him at my right hand, I will not be shaken....

> You make known to me the path of life;
> you will fill me with joy in your presence,
> with eternal pleasures at your right hand.
> (Ps. 16:8, 11)

If you watch your friends and classmates, you will likely observe a constant pursuit of fun and pleasure. Many teens seem to only look forward to the next outing, party, or weekend. They live waiting, hoping, and planning for the next "good time."

What does God's Word say about pursuing such pleasures? Yes, God wants you to have fun and enjoy life. Fun is not inherently a bad thing, but the pursuit of it can become all-consuming. But what about the worldly pursuits of pleasure that surround you? Are there any hazards involved in seeking happiness solely for its own sake?

In the big picture, we need to keep in mind that God has something more satisfying for us than the quickly passing pleasures of this life. The big picture question is not, "Did you have fun today?" It has to do with weighty matters, such as, "Did you help anyone today?" "Did you serve God?" "Were you compassionate?"

Eric Liddell understood the bigger picture of life and its fulfillment. We are wise to remember the testimony of his well-lived life:

- God's path of life
- The joy in His presence
- Satisfaction from using our gifts in serving others
- God's everlasting pleasures

Pastor John Piper once wrote, "The greatest hindrance to worship is not that we are a pleasure-seeking people, but that we are willing to settle for such pitiful pleasures."[12]

DISCUSSION STARTERS

1. What is your understanding of the *bigger picture* mentioned in today's reading?
2. Are you deeply assured of God's love for you? If not, what is getting in the way?
3. What does God's love for you mean, and how might it impact the use of the gift of your sexuality?
4. Can you explain what David meant by "eternal pleasures" in Psalm 16:11?

DAY 6
GOD'S PLAN FOR SPIRITUAL FREEDOM

President George W. Bush, in his 2003 State of the Union Address, pronounced, "Americans are a free people who know that freedom is the right of every person and the future of every nation. The liberty we prize is not America's gift to the world; it is God's gift to humanity."[13]

God wants us to live with freedom. We are blessed in our country to live with the freedoms we enjoy each day. Sadly, many are in bondage to addictions such as alcohol, drugs, pornography, and video games.

Jesus said, "Then you will know the truth, and the truth will set you free" (John 8:32). He also said, "Very truly I tell you, everyone who sins is a slave to sin. Now a slave has no permanent place in the family, but a son belongs to it forever. So, if the Son sets you free, you will be free indeed" (John 8:34–36).

Are you walking in freedom with God's plan for you relationally and sexually? Many teens are not. Josh McDowell has spent many years supporting pastors, youth workers, and parents in their efforts to pass on their faith to the next generation. However, he believes the fingertip access to internet pornography is having a destructive impact on young people. It is hindering receptivity to biblical values by distorting young people's views of sexuality and the Christian faith.

Josh McDowell Ministries hired the leading research

organization, Barna, to take on the challenge. The goal was to research the magnitude to which pornography has invaded Christian families and the church and to clarify its impact in detail. Studying pornography usage in the church is very difficult because the church has been disturbingly silent on sexual topics.

The church has a strong stigma attached to porn use. Those caught in its grip are much too afraid and ashamed to come out and ask for help. Here are critical findings from the Barna study *The Porn Phenomena* reported by Focus on the Family:

> For instance, the cavalier attitude toward pornography among the younger generations was alarming (32 percent say viewing porn is "usually or always wrong" compared to 56 percent who say not recycling is "usually or always wrong"). Usage among women also challenged some of our common assumptions about the gendered use of porn (56 percent of women 25 and under seek out porn). And the age at which young people encounter porn was much earlier than we imagined, with 27 percent of young adults ages 25–30 first viewing pornography before puberty.[14]

Every believer needs the daily reminder that our identity is not that of a slave but a son or daughter of God. The Lord has freed us from the power and the punishment of sin. We need to receive and appropriate God's grace to live free and fulfill our destiny. Paul wrote,

> Don't you know that when you offer yourselves to someone as obedient slaves, you are slaves of the one you obey—whether you are slaves to sin, which leads to death, or to obedience, which leads to righteousness? But thanks be to God that,

> though you used to be slaves to sin, you have come
> to obey from your heart the pattern of teaching
> that has now claimed your allegiance. You have
> been set free from sin and have become slaves to
> righteousness. (Rom. 6:16–18)

Bill turned away from the pressure of his friends to vape. (Please remember that all real identities have been carefully concealed and protected throughout this book.) Jack didn't give in to the temptation to view pornography on his computer. Susan didn't surrender to her boyfriend's repeated efforts to go too far on their date. That is freedom. Real freedom is the power to say *no* to sin and *yes* to what pleases God.

There is a battle raging all around us. Our calling is to be sexual freedom fighters in an overly sexualized world. We must know that we can be free—it is attainable with God's help. It will require some effort on our parts to "renew our minds" (Rom. 12:2). Ultimately, it can only be completed by the supernatural power of God's grace as we yield ourselves to His Spirit.

Freedom is like a two-sided coin. Breaking free from the chains of lust and masturbation is only one side of the coin. Freedom is not just *from* something. It is also freedom *toward* something, and that is the other side of the coin. You can say *yes* to your true spiritual identity and the desires of your heart. The Bible calls this self-control.

One teen commented to his youth pastor, "I was surprised by what happened when I quit the lust and masturbation. God started to work on me in some deep issues in my heart. I am alive now more than ever before."

God desires to do more for you than provide the strength to keep from lust and masturbation. He wants you to be free, of course, from those things. More importantly, He wants to empower you to enjoy healthy relationships and holy sexuality according to His design.

DISCUSSION STARTERS

1. What did you learn from the study on *The Porn Phenomena*?
2. Are you walking in the freedom of a son or daughter of God? If not, what keeps you in bondage?
3. What can you do to "renew your mind" daily?
4. What do you think are the most essential things needed to be true to your spiritual identity?

DAY 7
PRACTICAL HELP TO OVERCOME MASTURBATION

We have already said that there are differing viewpoints on the issue of masturbation. Many Christians have debated the issue. One expert will say that it's wrong, and another one will say it's perfectly fine.

We have tried to represent a balanced perspective throughout the daily readings. The Bible doesn't even use the word *masturbation*, so we want to be careful about what conclusions we draw. Can we know the truth on this matter? Yes, we can. God's Word does deal with the issue and tells us everything we need to know. Scripture speaks to the danger of lust and reveals an accurate view of sex.

God wants us to see the bigger picture. Masturbation doesn't matter to God because it involves our genitals, but because it affects our hearts. God's desire, above all else, is that our hearts be committed to Him. In Deuteronomy 6:5, we read, "Love the Lord your God with all your heart and with all your soul and with all your strength."

It is widely accepted that there are biological realities involved with lust and masturbation. God did make us sexual creatures with bodies hardwired to desire stimulation and sexual pleasure. A specific physiological component is undeniable. A guy's body produces semen that at some point has to be released. Teen males who don't masturbate will have wet dreams; the semen releases during sleep.

Many women have the experience of having what is called nocturnal orgasm. Women wake up "sexually aroused and sometimes even have a spontaneous orgasm."[15] We are all sexual beings. The nocturnal orgasm is natural and likely God's way of releasing sexual tensions, just like wet dreams for guys.

It may seem in some sense that masturbation is natural. However, *natural* doesn't necessarily mean *good*. We live in a fallen world, and we have all been impacted negatively by sin. Natural desires may quickly become sinful cravings.

Some Christians have argued that they can masturbate without lusting. They say that they merely have a physical release without sexual thoughts or fantasy. We cannot judge the intent or heart of another person. However, it is highly questionable that most men and women will make this argument. Be honest with yourself. Can you masturbate without the presence of lust?

Let's say that it was possible to masturbate without lust. Paul stated, "'I have the right to do anything,' you say—but not everything is beneficial. 'I have the right to do anything'—but not everything is constructive" (1 Cor. 10:23). You alone can make this decision. John Maxwell offered these wise words, "Life is a matter of choices, and every choice you make makes you."[16]

Is your choice regarding masturbation helping you to become the person God wants you to be relationally and sexually? Alternatively, is it creating a lifestyle built on a self-centered view of sex? Is sex becoming solely about your pleasure, your body, and your orgasm? The natural tendency and direction of sin is a self-focused pleasure. Self-absorption leads to an isolated experience that reinforces a view of life rooted in self-gratification.

If you would like to break free from this pattern, the first step is to renew your understanding of God's plan. You understand that your body belongs to God (Rom. 12:1), including your sex organ. Sex is a blessing from God for you to protect and save for marriage.

Overcoming lustful masturbation begins with a commitment to renewing your mind. You can also take some practical steps to change your habits. Here are some best practices for you to consider:

- Memorize key scriptures. Romans 12:2, Philippians 4:8, and Psalms 51:10 are excellent places to start.
- Meditate on this affirmation as you go to sleep: "Abba Father, I belong to you."
- Share your struggle with a trusted friend. Talking with a parent, youth pastor, or trusted friend is a great way to experience victory.
- Start the day by reading God's Word and praying. Your mind controls your sexual arousal. Your most important sex organ is your mind. So begin the process of transforming your mind (Rom. 12:2). Getting scriptures into your head and heart is essential.
- When tempted, redirect your thoughts to something else (exercising, shooting a basketball, listening to Christian music, and going for a walk).
- Work on victory only one day at a time. The "one day at a time" philosophy has benefits. It can keep you grounded in the present—that holy moment when God can be known.
- Never think about getting the victory for the rest of your life.
- Thank Him for making you a sexual being and ask Him to help you control yourself so you can enjoy sex in its proper context. The psalmist said, "I praise you because I am fearfully and wonderfully made; your works are wonderful, I know that full well" (Ps. 139:14).
- If you yield to the temptation, confess it as soon as possible— don't dwell on it. You will feel guilty because you have given in to your flesh and obeyed its desires, but don't keep punishing yourself about it. Scottish pastor Robert Murray McCheyne offered this helpful statement, "For every single look at yourself, take ten looks at Christ."[17]

As you do these things, lust will lose its hold on your life. If you slip, trust that God will help you. He understands that change takes time and effort. The goal is not perfection but rather progress. Don't give up. Stay the course. Remember, as Paul says, "I can do all things through him who gives me strength" (Phil. 4:13).

DISCUSSION STARTERS

1. What do you understand about the "biological realities" of the human body?
2. Can someone masturbate without becoming attached to lustful thinking or images? What about you?
3. Do you want to stop masturbation in your life? If so, what steps will you take?
4. What can you do to overcome the times of temptation?

WEEK TWO
WHAT THE SCRIPTURE SAYS

DAY 8
THE FAITHFULNESS OF GOD

Many teens struggling with sexual lust feel overwhelmed. Bill told his counselor, "I have battled with porn and masturbation for so long that I have given up. I promised myself so many times that I would stop. I don't believe I can ever do it!" Hold on to that statement, and we will come back to it.

A dad lifted his son, then about six years old, and placed him on the top of the slide. The boy was easily four feet from the ground. The dad held out his arms and shouted, "Go ahead! Jump and I will catch you." The boy looked down and paused. "Trust me, son! I'll be there for you." The lad gazed into the face of his father and then jumped. What happened next is hard to believe, but the dad dropped his arms and stepped back. The little boy landed on the hard ground and cried in pain. He was shocked and hurt. "There," said the dad. "This is to teach you an important lesson—you can never trust anybody, not even me. Don't forget it."

The boy never did forget what happened that day. He never did feel safe with his dad after that traumatic experience. Is it any wonder then that some think of God as a father who cannot be trusted?

Long ago, Moses wrote, "God is not human, that he should lie, not a human being, that he should change his mind. Does he speak and then not act?" (Num. 23:19). Moses affirmed that God is faithful and dependable in loving His children—not like the father about whom we previously learned!

Moses, the great leader and lawgiver, told us that God is not someone who fails to keep His word. Hear the confidence in his voice: "Know this: God, your God, is God indeed, a God you can depend upon. He keeps his covenant of loyal love with those who love him and observe his commandments for a thousand generations" (Deut. 7:9 MSG).

Absentee dads are a primary societal concern today. According to the US Census Bureau, 19.7 million children, more than one in four, live without a father in the home. Consequently, there is a father factor in nearly all social ills facing America today (US Census Bureau, 2017).[18] The data represent children living without a biological, step, or adoptive father. These are children whose dads are not there when there is a need. However, that is not true of God, whom scripture calls Abba Father.

If you are to understand the importance of your relation to Abba Father, it is helpful to learn about the strength of a biblical covenant. In Old Testament times, people made covenants with one another. These covenants are very similar to the legal contracts we use today; however, there is one notable difference. One of the agreements was established between two equals. The other covenant was negotiated between a mighty Sovereign and a lesser subject with little power.

That's the sort of covenant God makes with us—He is Sovereign, and we are weak with limited resources. His bond is one that cannot be broken down. Moses calls Him "the faithful God" and portrays His declarations as a "covenant of love." Throughout the scriptures, the loving Father cares for and wants to bless His children. The New Testament calls this *grace*—God wants to bless because you are His beloved child.

God is dependable in keeping covenant with His children, said Moses, for a thousand generations. In Exodus 34:4–7a, we read,

So, Moses cut two tablets of stone just like the originals. He got up early in the morning and climbed Mount Sinai as God had commanded him, carrying the two tablets of stone. God descended in the cloud and took up his position there beside him and called out the name, God. God passed in front of him and called out, "God, God, a God of mercy and grace, endlessly patient—so much love, so deeply true—loyal in love for a thousand generations, forgiving iniquity, rebellion, and sin." (MSG)

Keep in mind that a generation in the Bible usually is forty years, and that means then that a thousand generations would be forty thousand years. That is a long time! Moses is clearly saying that we can count on God all during our earthly lives and beyond to honor His promises. When life or others hurt us, Moses proclaims you can rely on God to be there for you.

Deuteronomy 33:27 says, "The eternal God is your refuge, and underneath are the everlasting arms. He will drive out your enemies before you, saying, 'Destroy them!'" His everlasting arms are beneath you, and He will lift you from the low times and put your feet on the solid rock. Could lust be among the enemies God will help us to overcome?

Remember, "God is not human, that he should lie, not a human being, that he should change his mind. Does he speak and then not act? Does he promise and not fulfill?" (Num. 23:19). You can count on a loving Father who sent His Son to reveal His faithfulness and steadfast love.

We are sometimes told in the church that we need a certain amount of faith before God fulfills a promise, that perhaps if we just believed harder, our prayers would be answered and maybe even sometimes a miracle might happen. It is no wonder that we feel it is our fault when we haven't seen a breakthrough.

However, 2 Timothy states plainly, "If we are faithless, He remains faithful, for He cannot disown Himself" (2:13). God's faithfulness makes us want to shout "Hooray!" How often can we feel so defeated by our lack of faith when facing a huge problem or crisis? The fact that the faithfulness of God is in no way dependent on you and me is such a burden lifted. We can just let God be God.

Considering all this, it is so important that we know His promises. When you see something in scripture, you can claim it as your own and feel hope rise. God didn't write the Bible for one person. He wrote it for us all, and all the promises are *yes* and *amen* for those in Christ today.

Here are a few of the promises that God makes us in the Bible:

- "The LORD will fight for you; you need only to be still." (Exo. 14:14)
- "The LORD himself goes before you and will be with you; he will never leave you nor forsake you. Do not be afraid; do not be discouraged." (Deut. 31:8)
- "But those who hope in the LORD will renew their strength. They will soar on wings like eagles; they will run and not grow weary, they will walk and not be faint." (Isa. 40:31)
- "Therefore, I tell you, whatever you ask for in prayer, believe that you have received it, and it will be yours." (Mark 11:24)
- "Believe in the Lord Jesus, and you will be saved—you and your household." (Acts 16:31)
- "And we know that in all things God works for the good of those who love him, who have been called according to his purpose." (Rom. 8:28)
- "And my God will meet all your needs according to the riches of his glory in Christ Jesus." (Phil. 4:19)

Let's go back to Bill at the beginning of this daily reading. We want to encourage him and ourselves with the many promises that God has spoken. Let's tell ourselves, "It's true—we cannot be sexually pure alone! The key is to take hold of the promises and believe He will empower us to do it. This is where knowing His character comes into play the most."

Now, knowing someone's character takes time. It involves ups and downs, waiting, and answering. May you increase in time to intimately know He who is faithful!

DISCUSSION STARTERS

1. What do Numbers 23:19 and Deuteronomy 7:9 mean to you?
2. Which one of the Bible promises means the most to you?
3. What does it suggest to you that "God is faithful"?
4. Moses delivered the Ten Commandments to God's people. What are the promises that come to God's people for following His commandments?

DAY 9
SEX IS GOD'S GIFT

Let's be clear about one thing: God created us as sexual beings. He made us male and female—and it is a good thing! God is not anti-sex; in fact, He created sex! It is His gift to His children.

The surprising truth is that God purposed in His heart to give us the gift of sex. God designed sexual intimacy as a gift to His children—and more than merely a means of reproducing human life. God also intends it as a way of giving and receiving physical pleasure as it grows out of the spiritual and emotional oneness in marriage. How brilliant!

We can go back to the Creation story and see that God purposed for us to experience sexual intimacy within the context of marriage. The Lord God said: "It is not good for the man to be alone. I will make a helper suitable for him" (Gen. 2:18). God intended for a man and a woman to be together. Marriage is a miracle from the mind and heart of God!

Do you realize that the first miracle God performed was the gift of marriage? God gave Adam the gift of Eve. When God presented Eve to Adam, Adam responded, "This is now bone of my bones and flesh of my flesh; she shall be called 'woman,' for she was taken out of man" (Gen. 2:23). Adam's first response was to declare the desirability he felt for Eve as well as the strong draw he felt toward her physically.

There can be no mistake that Adam uses real physical terms to express their bond and union—"bone of my bones and flesh of my flesh." An instant, permanent, physical connection existed between them, and it was placed there by God Himself, on purpose. So you're not weird when you feel that same attraction. You're merely operating in the way that God designed you.

However, God intends that this attraction ultimately links with a lifelong commitment. It leads to a marriage relationship based on a covenant that the man and woman make to each other before God: "For this reason, a man will leave his father and mother and be united to his wife, and the two will become one flesh" (Eph. 5:31). How can two unique individuals become one flesh? It happens through the promise and covenant of the man and the woman when they commit to and receive the marriage relationship as a gift from God.

Sex came from God, and God gives good things to His children. It's potent, intimate, transformative, and exhilarating. It involves every facet of a person's mind, heart, and body. It requires trust, tenderness, patience, and understanding. Sex is sacred because God created it. We are the ones who pollute sex when we engage in it outside of marriage. The results can be quite harmful and destructive.

Premarital sex can be a distressing experience for teens. Many sexually active teens say they wish they had waited. Fifteen-year-old Hannah explained that she began a physical relationship with her boyfriend, Steve, during her sophomore year of high school, even though "it felt embarrassing and weird." However, Hannah went along, and by the beginning of her junior year, she reluctantly gave in to his constant pressure. "I had always told my parents I would wait until I was in love and married," she said. "But Steve kept asking. Afterward, I thought, 'What did I do? Am I out of my mind?'"

Tim Gardener declares a powerful truth about sex in this statement: "It is both sacred and polluted, holy and desecrated. Its sacredness is based on its essence, which comes from God. Sex is holy because God created it to be holy."[19] We hurt ourselves and others whenever we act outside of God's intention and purpose for sex.

It's no great secret that teens who regularly view pornography live with deep feelings of shame. Humiliation and sexual sin always go hand in hand. In fact, this toxic emotion is most frequently one of the underlying psychological conditions that lead to addiction.

Shame is often a primary contributor to compulsive behavior. It is a heartrending emotion and leaves you feeling permanently ruined, broken, and unworthy of love. These feelings can, in turn, lead to severe anxiety, despair, anger problems, and lifelong difficulties with intimacy and relationships.

The shame identified here doesn't come from God and reveals a false understanding of our true spiritual identity. In comparison, we get a fabulous hint from Brennan Manning of the love of God revealed in Jesus Christ. He writes, "With a strong affirmation of our goodness and a gentle understanding of our weakness, God is loving us—you and me—this moment, just as we are and not as we should be. There is nothing any of us can do to increase his love and nothing we can do to diminish it."[20]

Shame is a gnawing awareness of our defects rather than the grace of God. Jorge, age eighteen, couldn't handle those toxic feelings anymore. Finally, he told his parents about the pornography and online contacts. His parents found a counselor, and Jorge explained to him, "After a few months of looking at porn, the masturbation, and the sexual messaging, I knew I was heading for disaster. I hated who I had become, and fear gripped me. Where was I going to end up? I couldn't see my girlfriend except as a sex toy, and she ended our relationship. I was trapped, desperate, and ashamed. I wanted to feel connected to God again."

Jorge found the following steps very important for regaining freedom from sin and shame. First, he acknowledged his struggle and feelings of guilt. There was no way to get better by continuing to judge himself. He realized that God forgave him, so he accepted

God's forgiveness. Second, he started to change some of his shame-based thinking. Jorge became increasingly aware of his spiritual identity. Third, he knew that he wasn't alone, and others fought the same battle with sexual temptation. Fourth, he reached out for help from his parents and therapist.

God wants you to experience the joy and freedom of healthy sexuality within the relationship of marriage. If you have made bad decisions, God wants to help you just like He did Jorge to find freedom and life.

DISCUSSION STARTERS

1. Do you understand that sex is a gift from God? What does that mean to you?
2. Why do you think that sexual shame is so powerful in its impact and pain?
3. What do you think about the statement made by Brennan Manning that God loves us "just as we are"?
4. This daily reading focused a lot on the topic of shame. What do you think is the key to overcoming shame?

DAY 10
PRESERVING GOD'S GIFT FOR ITS INTENDED PURPOSE

Robert M. Poole reported in the *Smithsonian Magazine* of February 2008 about looting in Iraq.[21] US troops were engaged in overthrowing the regime of Saddam Hussein in mid-April 2003. At the same time, US troops were sent to protect Baghdad's Iraq Museum from looting on April 16. Unfortunately, the looting had already happened by the time of their arrival.

Here is more of the sad story. The museum was vacated on April 8, and the first of the staff came on April 12. With clubs in their hands, the crew returned to find that thieves had stolen an estimated fifteen thousand items, many of them rare and priceless antiquities: ritual vessels, heads from sculptures, amulets, Assyrian ivories, and more than five thousand cylinder seals.

The losses were staggering. "Every single item that was lost is a great loss for humanity," says Donny George Youkhanna, the former director general of Iraqi museums, now a visiting professor at the State University of New York at Stony Brook. "It is the only museum in the world where you can trace the earliest development of human culture—technology, agriculture, art, language, and writing—in just one place."[22]

In the cultural war for decency, pornography has created bases of operation in the homes and hearts of most Americans. The treasures of sexual purity, relational integrity, marital sanctity, and youthful innocence have been trashed and trampled underfoot. The losses are staggering.

Richard Foster made this remark about God's design for the treasury of sexuality:

> Our human sexuality, our maleness and femaleness, is not just an accidental arrangement of the human species, not just a convenient way to keep the human race going. No, it is at the center of our true humanity. We exist, as male and female, in the relationship. Our sexualness, our capacity to love and be loved, is intimately related to our creation in the image of God. What a high view of human sexuality![23]

Sex was God's idea, not the invention of Hollywood or the pornography industry. It was intended as one of God's greatest gifts to His children. We are to treasure the intimacy, beauty, and the enjoyment of it. Sadly, our increasingly pornographic culture is teaching us to trash God's original design. If we are not well established in our relationship with God, we may place ourselves in danger regarding our destiny as His sons and daughters.

The Whitson's adopted eight-year-old George as their son. He had been a ward of the state since the age of two and in at least a dozen different foster homes. Old patterns ingrained in his brain continued to gnaw away at his self-perception and shape his behavior. The Whitson parents loved George like one of their own biological children.

He ate every meal as if it were his last. George would pile as much food as possible on his plate and devour every bit of it. His parents encouraged him to taste his food and then swallow it, but he acted as if he might not get a next meal. His feelings of neglect and abandonment haunted him.

One day his adoptive mother walked into his bedroom and noticed a foul smell. She thought their dog had an accident. She looked carefully and discovered a tuna-fish sandwich hidden under George's pillow. It had been on the lunch menu four days earlier!

George's environment had utterly changed from lack to abundance, from abandonment to belonging, from insecurity to security. He had a new identity. He was now a member of the Whitson family. It would take him years to grow out of the old ways of thinking and acting.

Similarly, we are transitioning from our old identity to our new identity in Christ. We are now members of the family of God. Paul wrote, "The Spirit you received does not make you slaves so that you live in fear again; rather, the Spirit you received brought about your adoption to sonship. And by him, we cry, 'Abba, Father'" (Rom. 8:15). He also commented, "so that you may become blameless and pure, 'children of God without fault in a warped and crooked generation.' Then you will shine among them like stars in the sky" (Phil. 2:15).

We have a new father and a new family, but our minds have been programmed by this world of confusion and darkness. We are in the process of seeing ourselves more and more as belonging to Abba Father. As Paul said, "Do not conform to the pattern of this world, but be transformed by the renewing of your mind. Then you will be able to test and approve what God's will is—his good, pleasing and perfect will" (Rom. 12:2).

In the real world, intimacy and romance require the efforts of true friendship, genuine respect, and affection. That is why the world of lust and porn is a cheap and false substitute for the demands of authentic, loving relationships. So many people today are spiritually malnourished and socially isolated, indulging in the moldy morsels of lust, masturbation, and sexual images.

We would be wise to use the gift of sexuality following God's intentions. According to the Bible, the purpose of sex is multidimensional. Sex is a gift from God with the intent of procreation, physical pleasure, and intimacy in its many dimensions. Sexuality is the fulfillment of God's created order in marriage between a husband and wife.

DISCUSSION STARTERS

1. Can you describe in your own words the cultural battle for decency?
2. What does the high view of sexuality by Richard Foster mean to you?
3. What does the story of George illustrate regarding your struggle with being a child of God?
4. Can you embrace the idea that God is your Abba Father? What does it mean to you?

DAY 11
YOUR TRUE SPIRITUAL IDENTITY

Imagine a new Mercedes-Benz rolling off the assembly line. It is advertised as one of the most luxurious and powerful vehicles ever made. The battery has been charged, and it gives a spark when the ignition is turned. But it won't start. Why? Hold on to that question for a moment and read on.

Imagine a male aborigine is flown in from New Guinea to inspect this remarkable vehicle. When he looks at the car, he is very impressed but confused. He has never seen such a thing, and he wonders about its purpose. Why was it created?

He quickly notices the symmetry, the chrome, and the paint job. It is attractive to the eye, and he first thinks the purpose must be for the sake of beauty. As he sits in the bucket seat, he wonders if it might be like a small hut. When he turns on the headlights, he thinks the car is for light. Then someone fills the car with gasoline and starts it up, and the vehicle begins to move forward. Now the aborigine understands the real purpose of the vehicle.

The car was created to provide transportation. The body, with all its excellent features, can't move on its own. The engine by itself doesn't have any power of its own; its only purpose is to convert the gasoline into a usable source of energy. Then, and only then, can the car complete its original design.

We were fashioned by God to live in close fellowship with Him.

God created Adam and Eve spiritually alive. At first, they were in constant union with Him. They lived with freedom and joy—and without shame. Regrettably, one day, they rebelled against God and chose to live independently from Him. This did not change God's purpose. It remains the same, and He has made provision for our healing and restoration. Nothing can transport us into a full life except being filled with the Holy Spirit.

Let's discover in further detail how we can become whom God made. We must not overlook the truth of Paul's statement: "'For in him we live and move and have our being.' As some of your own poets have said, 'We are his offspring'" (Acts 17:28). Just as a car cannot operate without gasoline, we cannot become who we are and achieve our full potential apart from God.

Some people may not see it as an addiction, but Howard struggled with pornography since the day of his first exposure at age seven. By age eleven, he knew he was addicted and felt trapped, ashamed, and alone. For seventeen-year-old Howard, viewing pornography online had started very early, and its impact was extensive. In fact, he later came to realize that the kinds of pornography he observed had a traumatic effect on him. He shared the words that follow with his therapist:

> I felt like every day I was damaged, like there was something terribly wrong with me. I was able to keep it a secret for several years from my parents. Somehow, I blamed them for not stopping me and getting me help. I convinced myself that I had to take care of the problem on my own, and I didn't think I could ever tell someone. The stuff I viewed was very hardcore and violent. I withdrew from everyone. I was filled with darkness and depression. I finally had to get help and tell my parents what was wrong when I tried to kill myself.

After three months of therapy, Howard began to see himself as a worthwhile person. This didn't happen until he finally admitted he had a problem. Another key was that his parents were able to demonstrate unconditional acceptance. They took part in his recovery, and even now, their relationship is growing stronger.

His friends started to notice a difference in his life too. He was no longer in chains to lust, masturbation, and pornography. He began doing better in school, and there was a visible change in his countenance—he started smiling. He said, "I am experiencing real joy for the first time in my life. It was the secrecy and the lies that kept me in bondage and oppressed. There have been two huge discoveries. The first was the beginning of the change in my life—I confessed my dark secrets to realize that others really do love me. I can't make it alone. The second is the most important discovery, and it is my awareness that God really loves me. His love is more than forgiveness. It's the power to change."

Not long ago, Howard didn't believe God could ever possibly love him. After all, he saw God as distant, angry, and vindictive. He certainly thought he deserved punishment. His counselor spoke to him about his past wounds, destructive behavior, and the steps to freedom. More importantly, he learned about the healing that comes from the Jesus of Calvary.

Somehow, he could understand God by looking at Jesus. Then he experienced a new understanding of his spiritual identity. He started to see himself no longer as unlovable and worthless. Instead, he came to understand that God's unconditional love was the foundation of his worth and value. He decided to turn his life and will over to the care of God.

As long as we are in this world, we will continue to face temptation. It is not a sin to be enticed by the thought of doing wrong. Christ was "tempted in every way, just as we are—yet he did not sin" (Heb. 4:15). We sin when we knowingly give in to temptation, something Christ never did.

The enemy, Satan, is always at work trying to get us to live our lives independently of God, to walk according to the *flesh* instead of the *Spirit* (Gal. 5:16-23). Satan knows the precise buttons to push when tempting us. He knows your weak spots and your family history. He knows the ways you have been injured and wounded. With your past, he knows your vulnerability to sexual temptations.

You may have accepted Jesus Christ as your personal Lord and Savior, but this doesn't mean old habits will cease right away. Sexual strongholds are challenging to overcome. We are in a world of constant bombardment from sexually stimulating thoughts. Sex is used in the media to sell everything from beer to hamburgers. Any prior exposure to pornography or ungodly sexual activities only strengthens sexual strongholds in your life.

The only way we can find freedom is to know the love of God through Jesus Christ. In Him, we learn of our supreme worth and the remarkable capability of His transforming love! Brennan Manning put it this way: "My deepest awareness of myself is that I am deeply loved by Jesus Christ and I have done nothing to earn it or deserve it."[24] Thus, self-acceptance isn't a matter of positive thinking or modern psychology; instead, it is exhibiting faith in the grace of God.

Your identity is established in Jesus Christ, and He is the foundation of our victory. Nothing is more central than realizing what God has done for you in Christ and who you are as His child. Your actions and responses to life's circumstances are greatly influenced by what you believe about yourself. If you see yourself as a helpless victim of life or Satan, you will be in bondage to lies. However, if you see yourself as a dearly loved and accepted child of God, you will find hope to live a life of sexual integrity.

DISCUSSION STARTERS

1. What did you learn from the story about the Mercedes-Benz and the aborigine from New Guinea?
2. Can you know yourself and your design apart from the Creator?

3. What do you think Howard learned that changed his life?
4. Do you agree with the statement made by Brennan Manning that your true identity involves being "deeply loved by Jesus Christ"?

DAY 12
THE THREE OWNERS

As an American teen, you have been told that your body belongs to you. The culture says you can do what you want with it. Many teen publications openly and unreservedly promote masturbation. An underlying belief is that pleasure overrules your decision making.

The Bible says, "Do not conform to the pattern of this world but be transformed by the renewing of your mind. Then you will be able to test and approve what God's will is—His good, pleasing and perfect will" (Rom. 12:2). This passage applies to both adults and teens who are believers.

Dr. Douglas Weiss shares a powerful revelation called "The Three Owners" in his book *Clean: Proven Strategies for Men Committed to Sexual Integrity*. It will help you better understand what God's Word has to say on this subject. You may be shocked to learn this, but there are three owners of your sex organ. Your sex organ doesn't just belong to you—not like the world says.

The first owner is your Creator God. A notable scripture is Romans 12:1, which says, "Therefore, I urge you, brothers and sisters, in view of God's mercy, to offer your bodies as a living sacrifice, holy and pleasing to God—this is your true and proper worship." Our sexuality is one way we honor and worship God.

God desires for us to worship Him with our entire being—including our bodies. Let's make this as nitty-gritty as possible. We need to ask for God's permission before we make decisions about masturbation, looking at pornography, or engaging in premarital sex. If we submit to His leadership and guidance, we will find freedom and victory.

The next owner is most likely someone you have not yet met—your future spouse. He or she is the most precious gift you will ever receive from God except for Jesus Christ! Your spouse is the person you will promise to love, honor, and cherish.

There is something you urgently need to know about your wedding day. It's something that you don't ever want to forget. Dr. Weiss says this about the day of a person's wedding: "On that day, at the altar of marriage, a sex-organ transfer occurred [will occur]."[25] Truthfully, this is what the Bible teaches.

Your future spouse will have an exclusive claim to your sexuality. Here is what the Word of God says: "The wife does not have authority over her own body but yields it to her husband. In the same way, the husband does not have authority over his own body but yields it to his wife" (1 Cor. 7:4). Most people still understand that when you marry someone, you forsake all others.

Let's look at this from where you are right now. The person you are dating will be someone's spouse one day. You have no right to their sexuality. Now, when you marry one day, your sexuality and your spouse's will be bound together, according to the Bible. Because of this understanding, here are two interesting questions. How will you treat someone else's future spouse? How do you want some other person behaving toward your future wife or husband?

The final owner for us to talk about is you. Hopefully, you are convinced that your sex organ is not only yours—it belongs to God, your future spouse, and then you. Put a smile on your face and hear what follows. As a partial owner of your body, you have the freedom to use your sexual organ to do what a person does in the restroom. If you understand that you are under the authority of God, then you are not free to do what pleases you.

Another relevant passage of scripture is, "Do you not know that your bodies are temples of the Holy Spirit, who is in you, whom you have received from God? You are not your own" (1 Cor. 6:19). "Therefore, honor God with your body" (1 Cor. 6:20). When you consider the definition of *temple*, it becomes clear why we should think of our bodies in the same way. A temple is a place dedicated to worship.

Here are two conclusions we can draw from 1 Corinthians 6:19–20: first, because our bodies are temples, we are to place high regard on them. Anything that brings glory to God is valuable to Him, and what is worthwhile to God must be prized by us. Human life is irrefutably precious, but if we are not careful, we can take it for granted.

The meaning of our bodies as temples is enormous. It involves giving care to how we handle stress. We demonstrate respect for our temples by getting adequate sleep, exercise, and nutrition. There is also the crucial issue of healthy boundaries regarding how we permit others to treat our bodies. All these matters reflect our understanding of the value God has put on our temples.

The second conclusion is this: Because our bodies are temples, we are to keep them holy. The specific circumstance Paul speaks about in 1 Corinthians 6 concerns refraining from sexual sin. The immediate peril that lies behind immorality is the contamination that it brings to our bodies. Similarly, sexual immorality pollutes the soul—negatively impacting our minds, emotions, and will.

The critical thing in this discussion was well identified by Jeremy Taylor, who wrote,

> The Pharisees minded what God spoke, but not what He intended. They were busy in the outward work of the hand, but incurious of the affections and choice of the heart. So, God was served in the letter, and they did not much inquire into His purpose; and, therefore, they were curious to wash their hands but cared not to purify their hearts.[26]

If we are going to respect God with our sexuality, we must honestly believe in the regenerating work of Christ in our lives. We will need to ask for the Holy Spirit to give us the ability to say *no* to sexual sin and *yes* to a life of sexual purity!

DISCUSSION STARTERS

1. How does the idea of the three owners challenge the world's view of the body? Does it influence your way of thinking?
2. What are the implications of believing that your body first belongs to God?
3. What does it mean to you that your body is a temple of the Holy Spirit?
4. The Pharisees are mentioned in this daily reading in terms of their focus on the outward aspects of the law. What can you do to purify your heart regarding your sexuality?

DAY 13

WALK BY THE SPIRIT

In Galatians 5:16, Paul tells the believers to "walk by the Spirit." He adds, "So I say, walk by the Spirit, and you will not gratify the desires of the flesh." Sure. Easier said than done.

Is there any way we can be sure that our actions are Spirit-driven? We can be easily confused about answering that question. A reason it can be so complicated is that we sometimes convince ourselves we are living by the Spirit when we are not.

A life directed by the Spirit, in contrast to the person controlled by the sinful nature, has these qualities: "But the fruit of the Spirit is love, joy, peace, patience, kindness, goodness, faithfulness, gentleness, self-control; against such things there is no law" (Gal. 5:22–23). This is a very significant list of characteristics for an individual to pursue. How can we experience these qualities in our lives?

No one has it completely figured out, but here are two things that can help you to walk by the Spirit. First, there will always be harmony between the Spirit of God and God's Word. Study the Word of God. It is true and unchanging, its applicability is never-ending, and it is captivating.

For example, the word *love* has assumed new and multiple forms of meaning over the years. We speak about loving our favorite sports team, pet, or friend. Those are all different applications when applied to the sense of love, but none of them compete with the love of God. This is never more evident than when Jesus encounters sexually broken people. We see His preference for people often rejected and shamed by others.

As Jesus lived among us, He intentionally encountered people with sexual struggles. His purity brought sunlight to their darkness. He destroyed the grip of shame with His mighty grace, and there's an inspiring example found in John 8:1–11.

One day Jesus appeared in the temple courts, and a crowd gathered to hear Him. Some of the Pharisees and religious leaders brought a woman guilty of adultery. It was a trap to discredit Jesus in the eyes of the public. According to the law of Moses, she could be stoned to death for her sin. Jesus knew their evil intent, so He demonstrated the heart of God in an extraordinary account.

This story reveals an unforgettable and glorious portrait of God's love. Read the text below and delight in what it shows about God:

> But Jesus bent down and started to write on the ground with his finger. When they kept on questioning him, he straightened up and said to them, "Let any one of you who is without sin be the first to throw a stone at her." Again, he stooped down and wrote on the ground.
>
> At this, those who heard began to go away one at a time, the older ones first, until only Jesus was left, with the woman still standing there. Jesus straightened up and asked her, "Woman, where are they? Has no one condemned you?" "No one, sir," she said. "Then neither do I condemn you," Jesus declared. "Go now and leave your life of sin." (John 8:6b–11)

Some interpreters believe that Jesus wrote down the sins of the accusers. Jesus brings the Pharisees and religious do-gooders to conviction about their shortcomings and sins. They drop their stones and walk away—every one of them. Next, Jesus offers this woman His unconditional love and acceptance with the encouragement to turn away from her sinful ways.

It may be hard to grasp that this same Jesus Christ offers you the same unconditional love. The truth is, in Jesus, you can find acceptance, love, and freedom. To do this, no doubt, it will take faith. Brennan Manning is right in saying, "Genuine self-acceptance is not derived from the power of positive thinking, mind games, or pop psychology. *It is an act of faith* in the God of grace."[27] We must give Him a chance. This is the first and most crucial step in healing.

Reading the Bible is the best way to learn how to love with God-like love. The Spirit of God will always lead you to do what is in alignment with the Word of God. It will guide you to love those who are broken—just like you. The news gets even better!

Second, the Spirit of God will lead you to freedom. Maybe you have tried to fight off sexual temptation. Sometimes you are successful, but at other times you fail. How do you handle those times when you give in to temptation? Let's turn to an excellent example of someone who knows well what to do in the case of a fall.

Nick Vujicic is no stranger to personal hardship and physical disabilities. He was born without arms or legs and, in his early teens, thought about taking his life. As you might guess, he knows a great deal about falling—more than most of us. But he never stayed down. His philosophy is summarized in a Japanese proverb that describes his formula for success: "Fall seven times, stand up eight." Nick doesn't view failure as final. It's more of a procedure of trial and error that serves a real purpose. You learn something from each fall that assists you in improving in the future.

If you slip up, it's not a reason to throw in the towel. Instead, it means you need to acknowledge your problem, ask God for wisdom, and trust more in the Holy Spirit for overcoming power. If you humbly seek wisdom, you will move forward and grow. Nick personified the core of a winning outlook when he said, "No matter who you are, no matter what you're going through, God knows it. He is with you. He is going to pull you through."[28]

For there to be victory, you must believe in your heart that you are worthy of it. You are, after all, His beloved! Then you must act assuredly, according to His direction. Fortunately, Nick overcame his disabilities and despair to live an independent, abundant, and fulfilling life. He is a great role model for all of us. You can read more about him and what he calls his *ridiculously good life* in his book, *Life Without Limits*.

Nick learned just how much God loved him. He adds, "It's a lie to think you're not good enough. It's a lie to think you're not worth anything. The challenges in our lives are there to *strengthen* our *convictions*. They are *not* there to run us over."[29] What are your convictions regarding your worth and the purpose of God in your life?

Hopefully, you are growing stronger in your convictions. Convictions are firm and fixed beliefs that guide and strengthen our lives. Here are some possibilities:

1. It is possible to turn from a life of sexual sin to a life of purity.
2. The foundation for lasting change is the grace of Jesus.
3. Jesus can, will, and does set people free from the power of sexual sin.
4. Real change isn't a human method, program, or just trying harder, but rather a trusting relationship in Christ and following practices based on His work.

There is real freedom available to us in Jesus Christ. It is freedom from trying to be perfect and never hitting the mark and freedom from the burden of attempting to be something we are not—and freedom from the condemnation that settles upon us when we fail.

Paul's words ring a triumphant note: "Now the Lord is the

Spirit, and where the Spirit of the Lord is, there is freedom" (2 Cor. 3:17).

DISCUSSION STARTERS

1. What are two things to help you *walk by the Spirit?*
2. What do we learn about love from the story of Jesus' encounter with the woman caught in adultery?
3. Brennan Manning spoke of grace as involving *an act of faith.* Do you have such faith? If not, what would it take to get it?
4. What is one of your convictions regarding your value and worth?

DAY 14
GOD'S MODEL OF GRACE

There are times we see areas in our lives that we struggle with—areas that we wish could be different. It might be poor habits that have us discouraged. How does God want us to address those areas? Is there a way we can change and find freedom? Yes, with God's grace.

When you understand God's compassion, it can make a reliable and sturdy difference in your life. What do you imagine when you hear the word *grace*? A winsome definition is offered by Rick Warren: "What gives me the most hope every day is God's grace; knowing that his grace is going to give me the strength for whatever I face, knowing that nothing is a surprise to God."[30]

Jesus once met a person named Zacchaeus, a Jewish man hated by his people. Zacchaeus was a tax collector and worked for the Roman government, the enemy. He not only collected a tax, but he added a surcharge on top of it for his profit. The Jews considered tax collectors to be traitors and thieves. Zacchaeus was no doubt a hardened man, but then he met Jesus.

Because of a crowd, Zacchaeus had climbed a tree to get a better view of Jesus. When Jesus walked by the tree, He looked up and said something that got his attention. He didn't shout out and call him a thief and a traitor. Jesus said, "Zacchaeus, come down immediately! I must stay at your house today" (Luke 19:5). Jesus kept fellowship with Zacchaeus and honored him by going to his house. It changed Zacchaeus's life, and he repaid those he had cheated. That was grace in action!

God's grace is what we need most when we become aware of aspects of our lives that we know are wrong. Once we receive Christ into our hearts, we are declared His own, forgiven, and empowered by His grace. Freedom and transformation are in His grace. Therefore, it is so important to know what scripture says about God's grace.

Here a few encouraging passages that link grace with life-change:

- "And with great power, the apostles gave witness to the resurrection of the Lord Jesus. And God's grace was so powerfully at work in them all" (Acts 4:33).
- "... but grow in the grace and knowledge of our Lord and Savior Jesus Christ" (2 Peter 3:18).
- "And God is able to make all grace abound toward you, that you, always having all sufficiency in all things, have an abundance for every good work" (2 Cor. 9:8 KJV).

Have you ever thought about someone, *I hope they don't learn this about me?* Alternatively, you may tell a friend, "Please don't share this with anyone else." When we get into our relationship with God, we may wonder if He is like we are. We think that we need to hide a part of ourselves from Him. Not so! We cannot hide anything from God, anyway.

On another occasion, Jesus was invited over to the house of a Pharisee named Simon for dinner. The party was crashed by a prostitute who began washing the feet of Jesus with perfume mixed with her tears. The Pharisee was offended and said, "If this man were a prophet, he would know what kind of woman is touching him. And what kind of woman she is—that she is a sinner" (Luke 7:39). Jesus knew who she was, and He spoke words of forgiveness over her. So Jesus broke the customs of His day. He was not only touched by a woman with a poor reputation, but He spoke to her of forgiveness. That was grace in action!

We can experience grace when we approach Jesus in simple truth and humility. We cannot come into His presence when we are trying to hide or keep a secret. What the law could not do, the grace of Jesus accomplished! We read in Hebrews 13:9, "It is good for our hearts to be strengthened by grace." God will grant us strength and grace if we come to Him in honesty and humility.

Look at Luke 18:10–14, where Jesus told this parable:

> Two men went up to the temple to pray, one a Pharisee and the other a tax collector. The Pharisee stood by himself and prayed: "God, I thank you that I am not like other people—robbers, evildoers, adulterers—or even like this tax collector. I fast twice a week and give a tenth of all I get." But the tax collector stood at a distance. He would not even look up to heaven, but beat his breast and said, "God, have mercy on me, a sinner." I tell you that this man, rather than the other, went home justified before God. For all those who exalt themselves will be humbled, and those who humble themselves will be exalted.

The healthiest people are aware of where they fall short, and instead of being defensive, they can say, "Lord, be merciful to me, a sinner." If we want to experience God's grace, we need to approach Him in truth and humility. James 4:6 says, "God opposes the proud, but He shows favor to the humble."

Some years ago, a teen shared his secret with his youth pastor. Zach, age sixteen, put it this way: "I was shy and lacked confidence in high school. When I got home from school, I got online to see my favorite porn fantasy girlfriends. If I were offline very long, I would get anxious and depressed. I couldn't focus at school, and

I stopped sleeping. I watched porn and masturbated late into the night. I lied for a long time about what was wrong, but my parents finally figured things out. I went into counseling, and it was very hard. It took me about nine months to get my life back. But God's grace helped me to get through it."

In Romans 5:20, Paul gladly announces, "Where sin abounded, grace abounded all the more." God's grace is available, but we must put our trust in Him. The apostle Paul said there is absolutely one inescapable condition that must be met if grace is to change us, and that is believing in God's loving-kindness in our hearts (Rom. 10:9–10). We must respond to God with trust and believe He will act as our loving Father.

He will receive you just as you are, but He won't leave you that way. John Powell said this: "We think we have to change, grow, and be good in order to be loved. But rather we are loved, and we receive His grace so we can change, grow, and be good."[31]

DISCUSSION STARTERS

1. Why do you think grace is so essential for real change?
2. How did Jesus' love change the life of Zacchaeus and that of the prostitute?
3. What has been your experience with God's grace? Has His grace helped you to change?
4. Jesus told a powerful prayer involving both a Pharisee and a tax collector. What did you learn from that parable about the importance of humility?

WEEK THREE
STRATEGIES FOR ALL WHO STRUGGLE

DAY 15
FREEDOM IN CHRIST

In many ways, we are all influenced by the culture in which we live. The culture today has many forces compelling us to conformity. We can identify the effects of the various media, the entertainment industry, educational systems, and political powers.

We cannot always reconcile the ways of the pop culture with those of the Gospel. John, the beloved disciple, commented, "Do not love the world or anything in the world. If anyone loves the world, love for the Father is not in them. For everything in the world—the lust of the flesh, the lust of the eyes, and the pride of life—comes not from the Father but from the world. The world and its desires pass away, but whoever does the will of God lives forever" (1 John 2:15–17).

This becomes very clear when taking notice of the pop culture and its influence. You have most likely heard the names of Elton John, Lady Gaga, and Ellen DeGeneres. They are prominent icons in pop culture primarily due to their wealth and fame. These people are looked upon as role models by many youths, and they have significantly impacted the culture's perspective on sexuality, especially regarding LGBT issues.

It is wise to view pop culture in light of the bigger historical picture. Otherwise, you may suffer from a minimal and narrow-minded understanding of yourself. This is a significant concern if you consider how pop culture overuses sexuality as a marketing tool. Much of pop culture is marketed toward teens and preteens. It is everywhere in the song lyrics, music videos, magazines, and television. This overexposure leads to pressure to become sexually active earlier and valuing sexuality over other aspects of life, such as the spiritual.

You might be curious to know that the idea of "teenagers" was created less than seventy years ago. It did not exist before World War II. The way it worked back then was that, first, you were a child, and then, you were a young adult.

Even eighty years ago, young people ages thirteen to seventeen would have lots of responsibilities on the farm or family business. They would be trained for employment, or domestic work, by age seventeen and married before the age of twenty. Most people were married and had become parents by their early twenties.

Generally, teenagers are not aware of the past, and this lack of knowledge can lead to limiting factors. The expectations of your peers can put you in a bind. Of course, there are big industries that market your fashion, music, entertainment, and technology. Knowing the human story can broaden your perspective and options.

This form of limitation or captivity is so prevalent today that most teens rarely even question it. When you are aware of human history and previous ways of living, it can free you to live more wisely and more compassionately. In other words, sometimes we can be so bound by our cultures that we lose sight of different ways of living and being. The goal is to live in a way that honors Jesus Christ.

Most of us want to be accepted and popular. That is especially true as a teen. It can feel devastating to be unwanted by friends. Lots of your energy may be spent trying to be cool and fit in. Moreover, if you are a follower of Jesus, that pressure may feel worse than rejection by friends. Hopefully, we want to please God more than our friends!

For many, fitting in is very important. However, what does it take to fit in? Here is a possible list:

- Phone
- Clothes
- Car
- Athleticism
- Hair
- Looks
- Video games

You have a brain. You probably know that it is superficial to live for such things. Sure, you want to be liked, but deep down, you know there are things far more critical in the long run.

Here is an illustration of what we mean. The following true story recorded by John Piper is a remarkable example of a teen named Jack Lucas:

> The year is 1945. World War II was still raging. Thousands of teenagers wanted to fight. The Battle of Iwo Jima was one of the deadliest—6,800 American soldiers are buried on that tiny island, many of them teenagers.
>
> Jack Lucas had fast-talked his way into the Marines at fourteen [in 1942], fooling the recruits with his muscled physique.... He stowed away on a transport out of Honolulu, surviving on food passed along to him by sympathetic soldiers on board.
>
> [At 17] he landed on D-Day [at Iwo Jima] without a rifle. He grabbed one lying on the beach and fought his way inland. Now, on D+1, Jack and three comrades were crawling through a trench

when eight Japanese sprang in front of them. Jack shot one of them through the head.

Then his rifle jammed. As he struggled with it, a grenade landed at his feet. He yelled a warning to the others and rammed the grenade into the soft ash. Immediately, another rolled in. Jack Lucas, seventeen, fell on both grenades. *Luke, you're gonna die*, he remembered thinking …

Aboard the hospital ship *Samaritan*, the doctors could scarcely believe it. "Maybe he was too … young and … tough to die," one said. He endured twenty-one reconstructive operations and became the nation's youngest Medal of Honor winner—and the only high school freshman to receive it.[32]

Knowing you are in war changes your perspective. If your family is being destroyed by sexual sin, any worrying about your clothes and your hair stops. There are more important things at stake. And we *are* at war. The enemy is stronger than the Axis nations of Germany, Italy, and Japan. The battle is daily. It is fought in every community, home, and life. The wins and losses of this battle lead to heaven or hell. The Word of God describes the battlefield in candid terms:

- "Put on the full armor of God, so that you can take your stand against the devil's schemes." (Eph. 6:11)
- "Fight the good fight of the faith. Take hold of the eternal life to which you were called when you made your good confession in the presence of many witnesses." (1 Tim. 6:12)
- "The weapons we fight with are not the weapons of the world. On the contrary, they have divine power to demolish strongholds." (2 Cor. 10:4)
- "Join with me in suffering, like a good soldier of Christ Jesus." (2 Tim. 2:3)

- "Dear friends, I urge you, as foreigners and exiles, to abstain from sinful desires, which wage war against your soul." (1 Peter 2:11)

Don't be like some teens who fail to see what is happening. They think they see reality by viewing the latest Hollywood movie or the most recent smart phone app. What is going on is that Satan is enchaining people or people are being set free by Christ. Moreover, Christ fights for the souls of people with the help of teen Christians.

But teenagers who are overly immersing themselves in the world cannot help fight. Teen *soldiers* know the familiar lies:

- "Everybody does it."
- "Sex is no big deal."
- "Oral sex isn't really sex."
- "Masturbating and porn are lesser sins than having sex."

Christ fights for the souls of people with the help of teen Christians. The devil wants you to believe his lies that life is all about comfort and pleasure now. However, our Abba Father and commander want us to know we are safe and stable in Him. Listen with your heart to your real identity.

- "Do you not know that your bodies are temples of the Holy Spirit, who is in you, whom you have received from God? You are not your own; you were bought at a price. Therefore, honor God with your bodies." (1 Cor. 6:19–20)
- "But you are a chosen people, a royal priesthood, a holy nation, God's special possession, that you may declare the praises of him who called you out of darkness into his wonderful light." (1 Peter 2:9)
- "The Spirit himself testifies with our spirit that we are God's children." (Rom. 8:16)

You were created for freedom, and conformity is not freedom. You belong to Jesus Christ. Let the world see in you that there is another kind of teenager made of humility and sacrifice, like Jack Lucas. You are encouraged, "Let no one despise you for your youth" (1 Tim. 4:12).

In fact, our God has sent a message to us on the battlefield that He will more than reward us—He will provide joy and eternal pleasures. Here, we can find in Him what the psalmist declared: "You make known to me the path of life; you will fill me with joy in your presence, with eternal pleasures at your right hand" (Ps. 16:11).

DISCUSSION STARTERS

1. What are your most significant pressures from the world?
2. What do you learn from the incredible story of Jack Lucas?
3. Do you think that Christ can use you?
4. Do you think knowing about *eternal pleasures* can help overcome sexual temptations?

DAY 16
WHY ACCOUNTABILITY MATTERS

The movie *Gladiator* starring Russell Crowe has a classic line in it. Russell Crowe plays General Maximus, the lead character and hero, who says to his soldiers as they are going to the battlefield, "Brothers, what we do in life echoes in eternity." Do you have an eternal perspective? Do you believe that your life is accountable to God?

Jesus taught that people are responsible for their actions and words and will be held accountable (Matt. 12:36). Are you approaching each day as if the Lord might return anytime now? Are you a believer who lives in a manner that there is no need to be ashamed (2 Tim. 2:15)?

We could rightly define sin as human nature bent on doing what we wish rather than what God desires for us to do. Alternatively, it is our propensity to be god rather than be held accountable to the one true God. This self-centered life leads to a gloomy condition of slavery to sin rather than joyful obedience to God.

God calls us to a life of healthy relationships and freedom. This freedom in Christ empowers us to live the abundant life (John 10:10). One of the significant ways this happens is through accountability relationships. God intends for us to encourage one another toward love and good works (Eph. 4:11–16; Heb. 10:24). This concept of biblical accountability with other believers promotes growth in Christ-like character through humility, honesty, and grace.

Accountability can happen in different ways. One is that you can take part in a weekly or small biweekly group with two to four Christian friends. You meet regularly for the community, Bible study, encouragement, prayer, and accountability. Additionally, this would be a local group so that you could enter one another's lives, share your problems, and equip one another for service.

Second, you can have a deep friendship with one person with whom you talk about spiritual things. It is advisable for this person to be the same gender as you. Accountability means finding that person who loves Christ and will love you unconditionally. This person should be

- someone you respect,
- someone you trust,
- someone you know cares about your spiritual development, and
- someone you can count on to see you through the eyes of Christ.

Also, he or she should be a person in whom you can confide and know that what is said will be kept confidential.

Another kind of accountability is a church family. Hopefully, your church is a place where you feel comfortable sharing your battles and asking for help. It should also be a place where the church members aren't afraid to question you in a loving, kind way. It's hard for this to happen unless your church is organized with community groups or you get involved in a small group. Accountability works best in close relationships.

Building these relationships often takes time and effort. It is not possible for those who are strong individualists or who have significant trust issues. There is nothing wrong with starting slow. Wisely, build the accountability relationship taking the time needed to construct it well. You will find that you both will benefit from such a relationship. Brothers and sisters in Christ rely on one another, according to the scriptures. Here are some examples:

- James 5:16: "Therefore, confess your sins to each other and pray for each other so that you may be healed. The prayer of a righteous person is powerful and effective."
- Galatians 6:1–2: "Brothers and sisters, if someone is caught in a sin, you who live by the Spirit should restore that person gently. But watch yourselves, or you also may be tempted. Carry each other's burdens, and in this way, you will fulfill the law of Christ."
- Ecclesiastes 4:9–10: "Two are better than one, because they have a good return for their labor: If either of them falls down, one can help the other up. But pity anyone who falls and has no one to help them up."
- Hebrews 3:13: "But encourage one another daily, as long as it is called 'Today,' so that none of you may be hardened by sin's deceitfulness."
- 1 Thessalonians 5:11: "Therefore encourage one another and build each other up, just as in fact you are doing."
- Proverbs 27:17: "As iron sharpens iron, so one person sharpens another."

The Bible illustrates very clearly that God meant for us to walk together. Even our Lord had His group of twelve to encourage Him, and of that group, He also had an intimate band of three with whom He shared more deeply. When Jesus sent out the advance team of seventy men to go ahead of Him, He sent them out in twos to places He would later visit (Luke 10:1). When the apostles went to proclaim the gospel all through the New Testament, they went in pairs. They needed one another. We need one another.

Consistent accountability can be a means of God's protection in your life. You are a new creation, and you have the Spirit's power.

It's no longer a surprise that when we want to do good, evil is close at hand (Rom. 7:21). Understanding that we are all on the same team (all sinners at the foot of the cross) means we can freely share with these close, trusted friends. Accountability allows us to confess our vulnerabilities, and in the process, we are prevented from stumbling.

The best-selling book *The 4 Disciplines of Execution* by Chris McChesney, Sean Covey, and Jim Huling speaks to this conversation. The authors state that the people who accomplish the most in life prioritize four things:

1. Focus on the Wildly Important
2. Act on the Lead Measures
3. Keep a Compelling Scoreboard
4. Create a Cadence of Accountability[33]

Goals require time, work, endurance, and dedication to achieve. And results often do not come without waiting on the Lord. You can quickly lose motivation in the process and give up. But everything changes when you build leverage with a system of accountability. To "be accountable," you need a clear goal and a willingness to let others help you achieve it. Jesus understood this principle, and this is how His church has continued for some two thousand years.

Achieving anything in life takes practice. Improving your relationship with God, building friendships, working out, eating healthy, and playing a musical instrument are rituals that progress with time. Whether you want to transform your habits, health, or a relationship, identifying the benefits and accountability can make it possible for you to reach your goals.

The American Society of Training and Development (ASTD) did a study on accountability and found these statistics about the probability of completing a goal in the following conditions:

- You have an idea or a goal: 10 percent
- You consciously decide you will do it: 25 percent
- You decide when you will do it: 40 percent
- You plan how you will do it: 50 percent
- You commit to someone you will do it: 65 percent
- You have a specific accountability appointment with a person you've committed to: 95 percent[34]

The point behind accountability also has to do with our purpose and mission. Answerability should also be a time to build each other up and encourage each other toward God's goodness and grace found in Jesus Christ. We remind each other who we are in Christ: accepted entirely, sons and daughters of the Highest, and created for greatness. We keep in mind that we can draw near to Him and His throne of grace. We can accomplish far more together for the sake of God's kingdom than alone.

DISCUSSION STARTERS

1. Do you think the words of General Maximus are right, that what we do "echoes in eternity"? If so, how?
2. How will you address the importance of accountability in your own life?
3. What do you think the several passages of scripture for today suggest are reasons for accountability?
4. What do you think about the ATSD study and its conclusions about accountability?

DAY 17
TREAT THE ROOT CAUSES, NOT THE SYMPTOMS

Imagine you have a crack in your ceiling at home resulting from a water leak. You could spackle over the break or replace a wet ceiling tile. However, would that fix the problem? Not so! You need to go to the source of the problem. When you do, you find a broken seal on the upstairs bathroom toilet above the ceiling crack. The seal needs to be replaced.

In another example, imagine that you go to an oncologist, and he diagnoses you with cancer and recommends chemotherapy. If you put a bandage on your skin, it wouldn't change the fact that you have a potentially fatal illness. This is a situation that requires treating the root cause. Your life is endangered!

Perhaps you struggle with emotional pain from your past or cannot relate to others. Maybe you have lots of trouble coping with your stress. You decide to find escape and release through masturbation and lust. Does that solve the problem?

On the contrary, superficial efforts to relieve the symptoms of a problem usually make things worse. The leaky ceiling drips more, and the ceiling stain expands. Cancer grows and threatens your life. Our interest in masturbation and lust deepens over time.

Fixing symptoms is taking the easy path. It doesn't require that much work on our part, and we feel relief very soon afterward. Unfortunately, this kind of "fixing" is fatally flawed. It doesn't resolve the problem and only makes the situation worse in the long run. Why do we hurt ourselves in this way?

First, we may not be adequately informed regarding the actual situation at hand. We incorrectly conclude that the symptom is nothing serious. And since this is our attitude, we feel we need to take no further action.

Then, even if we reason that there is something bigger happening in the background, we are still reluctant to act. This might be because the symptoms are not so severe, and we think that our situation is something we can handle.

You may also be delaying the discovery of the actual cause due to dread. You are really afraid to find out what is going on. Fear is often the most significant reason we are held back. If it's a health issue, you are perhaps afraid to face the unpleasant truth the discovery might reveal.

Still, the problem remains because you are not taking any initiative to find out the actual root cause. Wouldn't it be wiser and more compassionate to treat the root causes?

Dr. Harry Schaumburg wrote *False Intimacy*, and his book offers some real solutions for getting to the core of a relational problem. The culture today wants you to believe that you are made of biology and primal impulses. The goal of life is to satisfy you—so we are told. The author challenges you to do the following:

- Face yourself honestly without denial.
- Face your vulnerabilities and wounds.
- Recognize your need for change.
- Realize you cannot heal yourself and humbly turn to God.
- Rely on God to meet your needs.
- Confess your sins to God.
- Ask for help.
- Pursue healthy relationships.
- Realize that change is a process.[35]

We can each benefit from this wise counsel. When we turn away from sexual lust, we can choose a healthy pathway for authentic life change. We can find ways to solve problems and overcome our wounds. We learn to manage the power of our sexuality in a way that creates character and integrity. A humble, honest admission of need, turning to the Lord, and opening to other godly people are essential. It is a process worth all the effort.

Humility is our most potent weapon against sexual impurity. There is always a deeper root behind our lustful thoughts and behaviors. If we want to stop sexual sin, we must primarily address the heart. Moreover, the source of the problem here is not our sex drive. No, it's our egotism and selfishness.

What does the Bible refer to as the cause of sexual sin or brokenness? We can find it plainly in Romans 1:21–26.

> For although they knew God, they did not honor him as God or give thanks to him, but they became futile in their thinking, and their foolish hearts were darkened. Claiming to be wise, they became fools and exchanged the glory of the immortal God for images resembling mortal man and birds and animals and creeping things. Therefore, God gave them up in the lusts of their hearts to impurity, to the dishonoring of their bodies among themselves, because they exchanged the truth about God for a lie and worshiped and served the creature rather than the Creator, who is blessed forever! Amen. For this reason, God gave them up to dishonorable passions.

"Dishonorable passions" (vs. 26), which describes sexual acting out in all varieties, is a manifestation of humanity disconnected from its Creator. The real root of sexual sin is human arrogance.

C. S. Lewis called pride "the great sin." In *Mere Christianity*, Lewis said,

> According to Christian teachers, the essential vice, the utmost evil, is Pride. Unchastity, anger, greed, drunkenness, and all that, are mere fleabites in comparison: It was through Pride that the devil became the devil: Pride leads to every other vice: it is the complete anti-God state of mind.... It is Pride which has been the chief cause of misery in every nation and every family since the world began.[36]

The universal problem is pride, and we all suffer from it to some degree. God desires to forgive and restore us, but He cannot do that when we oppose Him in pride. He repeatedly says that He will exalt us if we humble ourselves.

Humility isn't in fashion in today's world. As Jonathan Edwards said, "We must view humility as one of the most essential things that characterizes true Christianity."[37] Even a glance at the Gospels reveals the most exceptional example of humility in human history: Jesus Christ. He came "not to be served, but to serve, and to give his life as a ransom for many" (Matt. 20:28).

Denial and superficial remedies make for less than a great life. We all want to look back knowing that we have dealt with our issues honestly. Humility will allow us to get started with our God-given destiny to learn, to grow, and to become more like Christ.

Humility is one of our greatest allies because it increases our hunger for God and opens our hearts to His Spirit. It creates intimacy with God because He dwells with those of "a contrite and lowly spirit" (Isa. 57:15). It imparts the aroma of Christ to those with whom we engage in life. Humility is a sign of greatness in the kingdom of God (Luke 22:24–27).

DISCUSSION STARTERS

1. Why is it important for you to treat the root causes?
2. What kind of real solutions does Harry Schaumburg offer? Do you see anything offered by Schaumburg as particularly helpful when it comes to real solutions?
3. What is the importance of humility in getting to the root problem of pride?
4. Do you think that it is important to be humble if you are going to overcome pride and have healthy relationships?

DAY 18
CREATED FOR GREATNESS

Did you ever play "king of the hill" when you were a child? There are many variations of this game. In the American Midwest, it is often played on bales of hay, or it might just be played on a dirt hill. It can be played with individuals or teams. The desire to be the last person standing is very tempting.

We recognize that there is a desire to be celebrated in us. Most people play it out over the duration of their lives. "King of the hill" becomes king of sports, king of academia, king of money, king of popularity, or king of technology devices. Striving for greatness has motivated a lot of people to do ungodly things and hurt others. False humility should not deter us from a desire for godly honor.

We need to establish a biblical perspective on this topic. Maybe it is not a bad thing to desire greatness. What if you were destined for greatness? This is not saying that you should knock people off the hill so you can get to the top. God has another way for us that is counter to the culture.

Nelson Mandela said, "There is no passion to be found *playing small*, in settling for a life that is less than the one you are capable of living."[38] That's a great quote to motivate teens on a basketball or football team. It's the kind of thing you want to hang on your refrigerator so you see it every day. And it has enormous implications for your spiritual life.

You face several real dangers—in "playing small," to go along with the crowd, and to hold back to ensure that no one notices you. But God placed His very Spirit within you. You are filled with the presence and the power of God. If you are faithful to your design by God, then you will stand out in some way and make a difference.

Think about the many biblical characters who were viewed as insignificant in the eyes of the world but who God used mightily:

- Moses, a stutterer, was used to deliver the Ten Commandments and lead the people of Israel to the Promised Land.
- Rahab, a prostitute living in Jericho, was used to contribute to the coming of the Messiah.
- Matthew, a despised tax collector, was used to write one of the Gospels.
- Saul, a former persecutor of Christians, became a powerful voice for the saving power of Jesus Christ, and his voice is still heard to this day.

Here is another story that illustrates God's great favor on us. It is the story of the much more famous Mary, the mother of Jesus. She was most certainly a teen and from a poor family. The angel came to her and told her that she would bear a child and that He would be the Son of God. The angel said, "Greetings, you who are highly favored! The Lord is with you" (Luke 1:28).

Mary's response to the angel was marked, understandably, with astonishment and fear. He bids her not to fear. That's easier said than done. She was not a married woman. Her pregnancy would bring many questions and public ridicule. Perhaps it would get worse. People frequently stoned pregnant, unmarried women in those ancient days.

Somehow Mary found it in her to say, "I am the Lord's servant. May your word to me be fulfilled" (Luke 1:38). This is a verse to consider and cultivate as a personal favorite. The reason Mary could respond in this manner was her deep understanding of her identity in relationship to God. She said, "I am the Lord's servant."

There is a pattern to imitate in Mary's affirmation to move forward with the great things God has planned for us. Notice her declarations and build a life of greatness on them:

> I am ...
> May it be to me ...
> I am blessed.
> I am highly favored.

Do you know who you are? Nothing that may be going on in your life right now can change God's view of you. Not only does God love you, but He likes you—and not because He's obligated to do so. It is because He wants to. You have His love and favor!

Jesus Christ inspired His followers to a life of greatness. Each of them lived way beyond what they had fathomed as possible. Jesus had told them it would be so: "Very truly I tell you, whoever believes in me will do the works I have been doing, and they will do even greater things than these because I am going to the Father" (John 14:12). This is most likely what Paul meant when he said, "Eye has not seen, nor ear heard, nor have entered into the heart of man the things which God has prepared for those who love Him" (1 Cor. 2:9).

Do you want everything God has created you to be? Why would you want anything less? It is not all clear yet what He has created you to be. Perhaps you will be a nurse, a doctor, a teacher, or a scientist. The possibilities are limitless!

Hopefully, you are excited just thinking about it. For sure, you are God's son or daughter: forgiven, redeemed, and loved with a forever love. You have the privilege to join with Him in bringing about His purpose on earth.

Every single one of us has been created with a unique combination of personality, passions, and talents so that we might do the specific work God created us to do. We are perfectly equipped to handle anything that comes our way if we would humbly pray for His power and act for His glory. The real danger for us was described by Pastor Steven Furtick: "The Enemy can't keep you from being who God says you are. But he can blind you from realizing who God says you are."[39]

Are you settling for a life spent playing small? There is no hope, no passion, and no glory in mediocrity. As we study the scriptures, it is easy to see that Christ is indeed highly passionate, all glorious, and the very essence of hope. If we are to live a life that looks like Jesus, we must reflect these same attributes in our own lives. We cannot glorify Him while avoiding our part within His plan. He is looking for a generation that will serve Him with devotion and integrity.

Live your life with passion and refuse to accept anything less than that for which you were created. This is no time for "playing small"; now is the time to declare that you will live large for the glory of God. No more settling for little things; you are a child of God, and you were created to do great things. Pastor Craig Groeschel says, "When you know who you are, you will know what to do."[40]

DISCUSSION STARTERS

1. Have you ever pursued greatness in unhealthy ways?
2. What is your understanding of the Bible's perspective on greatness?
3. Do you agree with the statement made by Pastor Craig Groeschel that you will know what to do when you know who you are?
4. A lot was said about Mary, the mother of Jesus, in this daily reading. What can you learn from her about greatness?

DAY 19
DEVELOP DISCIPLINED CHARACTER

Self-discipline is a character quality that shows up in every aspect of our lives. It is a habit, a practice, a way of looking at and living life. Successful people are well known for their self-discipline. It is atypical to find a person with self-control regarding sexual desire that doesn't exert similar control in other areas of life.

President Theodore Roosevelt wisely described the value of discipline in this way:

> The one quality which sets one man apart from another—the key which lifts one to every aspiration while others are caught up in the mire of mediocrity is not talent, education, nor intellectual brightness. It is self-discipline. With self-discipline, all things are possible. Without it, even the simplest goal can seem like the impossible dream.[41]

You can define discipline as establishing one's conduct on principle. For the Christian, it is also a life patterned after Jesus Christ and learning to love and honor Him. The disciplined follower stays focused on high-value priorities. They are not controlled by impulse, emotion, or pressure from others. Instead, they delay gratification for the achievement of long-term goals.

It turns out that a marshmallow can be quite revealing about us. Walter Mischel conducted a landmark behavioral experiment on deferred gratification at Stanford University in 1972. Delayed gratification is a person's ability to resist the temptation of an immediate reward in anticipation of a more significant benefit.

Mischel conducted his experiment with a group of over six hundred children. The boys and girls were ages four to six. Every child was asked to sit at a table in a room with no amusements and was given a single marshmallow treat on a small plate. The child was then told that he or she would be given an additional marshmallow for waiting several minutes. They would have to wait until the experimenter returned in about fifteen to twenty minutes. As expected, many children ate the marshmallow as soon as the researcher left the room. But of all those who tried to wait, about 30 percent were successful in delaying gratification and gained the additional marshmallow.

How did these children succeed at waiting? Mischel, Shoda, and Rodriguez (1989) state,

> ... those who were most successful in sustaining delay seemed to avoid looking at the rewards deliberately, for example, covering their eyes with their hands and resting their heads on their arms. Many children generated their own diversions: they talked quietly to themselves, sang, created games with their hands and feet, and even tried to go to sleep during the waiting time. Their attempts to delay gratification seemed to be facilitated by external conditions or by self-directed efforts to reduce their frustration during the delay period by selectively directing their attention and thoughts away from the rewards.[42] (pp. 934–935)

During the first follow-up study in 1988, Mischel made some fantastic discoveries. The kids had recently graduated from high school, and the differences among them were significant and noteworthy. Those who deferred gratification were more optimistic, self-motivated, and determined in the face of challenges. They could delay gratification in pursuit of their goals.

Children who were able to defer gratification were described by their parents as being more assertive, confident, and more academically competent than those who couldn't wait for a second marshmallow. In the second follow-up study in 1990, the ability to delay gratification was linked with higher SAT scores. Children who could wait for the second marshmallow scored an average of 1262 (out of 1800) on the SAT. Those who ate their marshmallow early had an average score of 1052.[43]

Self-discipline is the one quality that you can develop that will assure you of greater success, accomplishment, and happiness in life. Successful men and women are usually disciplined in their work. Self-discipline is so necessary that if you don't develop it, it will be impossible for you to achieve your fullest potential.

Too many people are swayed by the pull of instant gratification. People who lack control don't think about the long-term effects of their decisions. This is one reason why this is such a crucial skill to have in life. It allows you to choose from various options and overcome the obstacles that are in your path. It has been wisely stated, "Discipline is the bridge between goals and accomplishment."[44]

One thing that is different about Christian character is that we answer first and foremost to God. The "fear of the Lord" is the biblical language for it. Solomon said, "The fear of the LORD is the beginning of wisdom, and knowledge of the Holy One is understanding" (Prov. 9:10). Billy Graham described it as of supreme value, saying, "When wealth is lost, nothing is lost; when health is lost, something is lost; when character is lost, all is lost."[45]

The personal qualities of our character count the most with God. He considers our behavior based on what is in our hearts (compare Jeremiah 17:10; Deuteronomy 10:12). "The LORD does not look at the things people look at. People look at the outward appearance, but the LORD looks at the heart" (1 Sam. 16:7). According to the Bible, the word *heart* is used to describe our motives, innermost thoughts, and attitudes. God knows what is taking place inside our minds. He evaluates our intents and motivations (Heb. 4:12–13).

Christian character is lived out of reverence and love for God, as contrasted to merely pleasing ourselves. The starting place is the fear of God, but what it boils down to is the willingness to die to our selfish desires. Jesus Christ demonstrated this humility and character in the Garden of Gethsemane when he uttered, "Father, if you are willing, take this cup from me; yet not my will, but yours be done" (Luke 22:42).

Christ-like character involves sacrifice, and that is something our culture does not emphasize. That is something only humble faith can produce in us. We are called to be servants—not just a people of integrity, but servants. Jesus said, "For even the Son of Man did not come to be served, but to serve, and to give His life as a ransom for many" (Mark 10:45).

The apostle Paul reiterated much the same thing when he said, "Have the same mindset as Christ Jesus: Who, being in very nature God, did not consider equality with God something to be used to his own advantage; rather, he made himself nothing by taking the very nature of a servant, being made in human likeness" (Phil. 2:5–7).

Every time you are tempted to masturbate and lust, think "Marshmallows!" The capacity to make a disciplined choice will become useful in other parts of your life journey. It will undoubtedly have spiritual importance. Paul spoke about this candidly when he wrote in 1 Corinthians 9:24–27,

> Do you not know that in a race all the runners run, but only one gets the prize? Run in such a way as to get the prize. Everyone who competes in the games goes into strict training. They do it to get a crown that will not last, but we do it to get

a crown that will last forever. Therefore, I do not run like someone running aimlessly; I do not fight like a boxer beating the air. No, I strike a blow to my body and make it my slave so that after having preached to others, I myself will not be disqualified for the prize.

Pastor Tim Gardner writes,

A hard drive that is unplugged from its computer will never fully do what it was designed to do. Sex, unplugged from marriage and our spiritual selves, will never do what it was designed to do. The separation of our sexuality from our spirituality causes the sexual pain and evil that pervade our world. When engaged in without God by people without an understanding of the holy, sex becomes an object whose only purpose is biological sensation or procreation.[46]

The Bible defines the context for self-discipline and sex within marriage. Galatians 2:22 reminds us that self-discipline is a characteristic of the Holy Spirit and the natural fruit of our lifestyle. When you make wise choices with the gift of your sexuality, you reap the fruit of blessings, a wholesome lifestyle. When you fail to exercise self-discipline with this most precious gift, you experience much anguish and regret.

This self-discipline is really a form of freedom. Martin Luther once exclaimed, "The person who is most free is disciplined."[47] This freedom rooted in our relationship and followership of Jesus Christ will usher in what Nick Vujicic calls the "ridiculously good life."

DISCUSSION STARTERS

1. Do you agree with the statement made by Theodore Roosevelt about the significance of self-discipline?
2. What do you learn from Stanford University's Walter Mischel's classic behavioral experiments on deferred gratification involving children and marshmallows?
3. How does self-discipline regarding your sexuality reflect on your character and future?
4. What impact does your reverence for God have on your Christian character?

DAY 20

USE YOUR SPIRITUAL WEAPONS

The prevailing worldview today has removed spiritual warfare as a category. We are told it does not really exist, yet Jesus tells us differently. He said, "The thief comes only to steal and kill and destroy; I have come that they may have life, and have it to the full" (John 10:10).

Jesus bonded these two statements together for a reason. He says these statements in the same breath, and He has two primary aims. First, He wants you to know that God intends for you to experience life! That's good news. Second, He wants you to know that you are opposed. There is a thief, Satan, who comes to rob you of your God-given destiny. You will have to fight for your life and future.

We must make no mistake about it—we are at war, and we must arm ourselves for battle. John Eldredge put it his way: "I'm sorry if I'm the one to break this news to you: you were born into a world at war, and you will live all your days in the midst of a great battle, involving all the forces of heaven and hell and played out here on earth."[48]

In Ephesians 6:10–17, Paul gives specific advice about spiritual warfare. If we follow his advice, we will be able to protect ourselves and face challenges in life with confidence. He identifies the weapons God makes available but that we must employ. When Paul wrote the letter to the Ephesians, he wrote from personal knowledge about Roman soldiers as he spent time chained to one. He described himself as "an ambassador in chains" (Eph. 6:20).

This passage is essential to understand. In Ephesians 6:10–11 (The Message), Paul writes, "And that about wraps it up. God is strong, and he wants you strong. So, take everything the Master has set out for you, well-made weapons of the best materials. And put them to use so you will be able to stand up to everything the devil throws your way." The armor mentioned here is symbolic, and it is no less than Christ Himself.

Every believer knows Christ as Savior. The problem comes when we do not appreciate all our Lord brings with Him. In the battles of life, Christ is the answer. When it comes to sexual temptation, Paul reminds us, "Rather, clothe yourselves with the Lord Jesus Christ, and do not think about how to gratify the desires of the flesh" (Rom. 13:14). In other words, we are to be empowered by the grace and the weapons He provides for daily life.

It is possible to forget these pieces of armor, but it is wise to take them up every day. Let's look at each of them and note their significance. Paul is commanding us to put on the entire outfit of armor. Let's look at them one by one.

The *belt of truth* served two essential purposes for the Roman soldier. It held his weapons and equipment together. The Roman soldier also used the belt to bind his robe and gear to keep from tripping. This spiritual weapon refers to the Word of God, and especially to Jesus, who said, "I am ... the truth" (John 14:6). It is our dependency on Him that keeps us from tripping over the temptations and obstacles in the world. This belt of truth is demonstrated when our lives are characterized by honesty and integrity.

The *breastplate of righteousness* is a precious gift from God. We are told how this is made possible in 2 Corinthians 5:21: "God made him who had no sin to be sin for us, so that in him we might become the righteousness of God." We are made righteous because He has ascribed His righteousness to us. This is a gift of God's grace. This gift enables us to reign in life, and we are now viewed as royalty!

A breastplate was designed to deflect the blow of the Enemy. The righteousness of Christ protects us in the same way. We know that we are unconditionally accepted by Him, and this deflects the arrows of rejection by others. We no longer must perform to be esteemed God's beloved. At the same time, we want to live in such a way as to honor God.

The Enemy, Satan, will try to get us to accept his lies. He promotes lies like, "You are nothing," "God doesn't love you," and "You have no future." He comes at us with all kinds of attacks. The only way he can get through is if we agree with his lies and choose the wrong pathway—whether in anger, pouting, self-pity, or self-rejection. If we protect our hearts with the breastplate of righteousness, we understand the words of Brennan Manning: "How glorious the splendor of a human heart that trusts that it is loved!"[49]

Another piece of the armor is the *warrior's shoes* (Eph. 6:15). The soldier's boots had a thick leather sole with hobnails to serve as cleats. These were tied to the feet and legs with leather laces. These boots served three purposes: (1) to provide a firm footing, (2) to furnish protection, and (3) to enable mobility. Our spiritual shoes serve a similar purpose. They help us to see clearly the foundation upon which we stand and keep us moving.

The identity of the shoes is described as "the gospel of peace." *Gospel* means "good news." Paul described the gospel as the death, burial, and resurrection of Christ (1 Cor. 15:1–4). Our firm footing is the ageless message of Jesus Christ. This message proclaims, "It is for freedom that Christ has set us free. Stand firm, then, and do not let yourselves be burdened again by a yoke of slavery" (Gal. 5:1). There is but one gospel and one way to be saved and find real freedom: "Salvation is found in no one else, for there is no other name under heaven given to mankind by which we must be saved" (Acts 4:12).

The *shield of faith* (Eph. 6:16) can be understood by looking at other passages of scripture. King David wrote, "But You, O Lord, are a shield for me" (Ps. 3:3). God spoke to Abraham, saying, "Do not be afraid, Abram. I am your shield, your exceedingly great reward" (Gen. 15:1). We take the shield of faith when we trust in the Lord. This means that we are to live by faith. We also hold to the assurance that we are saved by faith in Jesus Christ. Paul wrote, "The life I now live in the body, I live by faith in the Son of God, who loved me and gave himself for me" (Gal. 2:20).

The test of faith comes on the daily battlefield of life. This is not a big surprise to us, and it does not alarm us. The Lord was tempted by the Enemy in the wilderness. When Paul wrote of this shield of faith, he was in prison. The Enemy will hurl his fiery darts, and they sometimes come as temptation. They come as accusations and lies. The wise teen always answers these attacks with the Word of God! John, one of Jesus' closest friends, explained how we can deal triumphantly with these flaming arrows used by the Enemy. "This is the victory that has overcome the world—our faith" (1 John 5:4) in Jesus Christ.

We are given a complete set of armor that is adequate to carry us through the battlefields of this life. Another piece of armor is the *helmet of salvation* (Eph. 6:17). This is our assurance of God's protection until the day He comes back. In 1 Thessalonians 5:4–9, the helmet is clearly defined as the "hope of salvation." We can keep our minds from being messed up by remembering that the Lord is in control and that He is coming again.

A final weapon mentioned is the *sword of the Spirit* (Eph. 6:17), and it is described as the Word of God. It is a command for us all as warriors to take what God has available. The offensive weapon God offers is His Word. The Word of God is to be used to attack our Enemy, Satan. The sword is not of human origin. He places it in our hands.

You may remember the story of King Arthur and his knights. King Arthur's fighting ability was his sword, Excalibur, and this special sword endowed him with extraordinary power. So it is with each believer. The sword of the Spirit offers us a weapon of unlimited potential.

You now have some basic strategies and tactics to help you win the war. More importantly, you have heard the rallying call to put on the full armor of God. You are getting more and more equipped to be a mighty person who lives and honors God!

God wants to grow a new generation of young men and women committed to purity. You can be a hero but only to one person. The story of your future spouse is the only one in which you can be a hero. It takes a lifetime of commitment, faithfulness, and love. A real hero steers away from sexual sin to protect and bless his or her family.

DISCUSSION STARTERS

1. What do you think of the statement made by John Eldredge that we are "born into a world at war"?
2. What parts of the armor do you most need?
3. How do you understand Jesus' statement in John 10:10?
4. What do the words of Brennan Manning mean to you, when he says, "How glorious the splendor of a human heart that trusts that it is loved"?

DAY 21
ENJOY A LOVE RELATIONSHIP WITH ABBA FATHER

Since we live in this world, we will continue to face temptation. It is not a sin to be tempted. Christ was "tempted in every way, just as we are" (Heb. 4:15). We sin when we knowingly give in to temptation, something Christ never did.

The Enemy is always at work trying to get us to live independently of God, to walk according to the *flesh* instead of the *Spirit* (Gal. 5:16–23). Satan knows the buttons to push when tempting us. He is aware of our weak spots and our family history. He knows the ways we are wounded and our vulnerability to sexual temptation and lust.

You may have accepted Jesus Christ as your personal Lord and Savior, but this doesn't mean old habits will cease right away. Sexual strongholds are challenging to overcome. We are in a world of constant bombardment from sexually stimulating thoughts because sex is used in the media to sell everything from clothes to hamburgers. Any prior exposure to pornography or ungodly sexual activities only strengthens sexual strongholds in your life.

The only way we can find freedom is to know the love of God through Jesus Christ. In Him, we learn of our great worth and the power of His love. Brennan Manning put it this way: "My deepest awareness of myself is that I am deeply loved by Jesus Christ and I have done nothing to earn it or deserve it. Self-acceptance isn't a matter of positive thinking or pop psychology; rather, it is having trust in the grace of God."[50]

Our identity is established in Jesus Christ. He is the source of our life and eternal life. Nothing is more important than realizing what God has done for you in Christ and who you are as His child. Your actions and responses to life's circumstances are greatly influenced by what you believe about yourself. If you see yourself as a helpless victim of life, you will be in bondage to lies. But if you see yourself as a dearly loved and accepted child of God, you will find hope to live a clean life.

The Enemy, Satan, wants us to believe that God doesn't love us. But the truth is only those who fail to turn to God end up missing out on His mercy. Jesus clearly shows us that God is love and accepts us. He is full of compassion. We can bring Him all our hurts, sins, and bad habits. And when we approach Him in brokenness and humility, God receives us mercifully and with the promise of His help.

Mercy is not getting what we deserve, and grace is being given what we could never earn or deserve. The apostle Paul writes, "For it is by grace you have been saved, through faith—and this is not from yourselves, it is the gift of God—not by works, so that no one can boast" (Eph. 2:8–9).

No words can describe the limitless gifts God lovingly gives to His children. The riches of His grace are incomparable. It can be so difficult for us to hear about and receive this love. Why?

We find it hard to believe in God's love because of how we feel about ourselves, deep down. Hear this: We cannot accept love from another human being if we do not love ourselves. This is no less true when it comes to allowing God to care for us.

One of the most shocking things in the church today is the dislike many followers of Jesus have for themselves. It may be surprising to learn, but many are more critical of their imperfections than they are of anyone else's. David Seamands wrote, "Many Christians ...

find themselves defeated by the most psychological weapon that Satan uses against them. This weapon has the effectiveness of a deadly missile. Its name? Low self-esteem … a gut level feeling of inferiority, inadequacy, and low self-worth."[51]

God loves just as we are—whether we like it or not. God calls us out of our hiding. Just as He called us into existence, He calls us out of self-hatred to step into His truth. Jesus says, "Come to me, all you who are weary and burdened, and I will give you rest. Take my yoke upon you and learn from me, for I am gentle and humble in heart, and you will find rest for your souls. For my yoke is easy and my burden is light" (Matt. 11:28–30). We are safe with Jesus. He wants to help us.

Did you know that in scripture, many different names are used to describe God? While all the names of God are essential, the name Abba Father is one of the most significant for understanding how He relates to us. *Abba* is an Aramaic word that can firmly be interpreted as "Daddy." It is the terminology young children used in the New Testament period to address their fathers. It indicates the close, intimate relationship of a father to his child, as well as the innocent trust a young child puts in his or her daddy.

It is life-changing to comprehend the full force of what it means to be able to call the one true God *Daddy* and what it means to be joint beneficiaries with Christ. Due to our relationship with God, we know He no longer deals with us as deserving judgment. We can approach Him, a holy God, as our Heavenly Father with both "boldness" (Heb. 11:19) and the complete "assurance of faith" (Heb. 11:22). We have that self-assurance because of the presence of the Holy Spirit giving "witness with our spirit that we are children of God, and if children, then heirs—heirs of God and joint-heirs with Christ, if indeed we suffer with Him, that we may also be glorified together" (Rom. 8:16–17).

There are many benefits in being an adopted child of God. Becoming a child of God is an incredibly great privilege and honor; it is the most awesome gift in all the universe! This adoption process changes our relationship and standing with God. He deals with His children in a different way than the remainder of the world. Being a child of God, adopted "through faith in Christ Jesus," provides the basis for our hope, the confidence of our future, and the inspiration to "live a life worthy of the calling you have received" (Eph. 4:1). Being children of the Lord God Almighty calls us to a life of freedom and hope.

As we come to understand the true nature of God as revealed in the Bible, we become amazed that He not only allows us but encourages us to call Him *Abba Father*. It is impressive that the holy and righteous God—the one who creates and sustains all things, the only all-powerful, all-knowing, ever-present God—allows sinners like us to call Him *Daddy*. When we come to understand who God is and how we miss the mark, the honor of calling Him Abba Father takes on a whole new meaning for us and helps us to understand better God's amazing grace.

The apostle Paul, in his letter to the Galatians, wrote, "Because we are children, God has dispatched the Spirit of his Son into our hearts, saying, 'Abba, Father!'" (Gal. 4:6). Here is one way to further illustrate the significance of *the Abba experience*. It is a story told by Brennan Manning, in his own words:

> Years ago, I related a story about a priest from Detroit named Edward Farrell, who went on his two-week summer vacation to Ireland. On a great day, the priest and his uncle got up before dawn and dressed in silence. They took a walk along the shores of Lake Killarney and stopped to watch the sunrise. Suddenly the uncle turned and went skipping down the road. He was radiant, beaming, smiling from ear to ear. His nephew said, "Uncle Seamus, you really look happy." "I am, lad." "Want to tell me why?" His eighty-year-old uncle replied, "Yes, you see, my Abba is very fond of me."[52]

Take some time to consider what the Abba experience means to you. Do you know God as your Abba? If this is something new to you, you are encouraged to ask God to help you experience in a real way the love He has for you.

Saying *Abba Father* is a powerful and life-changing affirmation. The apostle Paul understood this when he wrote, "The Spirit you received does not make you slaves so that you live in fear again; rather, the Spirit you received brought about your adoption to sonship. And by him, we cry, 'Abba, Father.' The Spirit himself testifies with our spirit that we are God's children" (Rom. 8:15–16).

DISCUSSION STARTERS

1. What lies has Satan used to put you in bondage?
2. Are you aware that Jesus Christ profoundly loves you?
3. Why do you think that Jesus started the prayer He taught us with "Our Father … " (Matt. 6:13)?
4. Will you affirm for forty days this statement, "Abba Father, I belong to you," and see how it changes things for you?

WEEK FOUR
GOD'S DESIGN FOR SEX

DAY 22
SEX IS SACRED

What does it mean when we say sex is *holy*? A story in the Old Testament helps us answer this question. The concept of holiness is at the heart of God's identity, which we will encounter when we meet Him.

Moses was in the desert one day when he approached a burning bush with considerable apprehension because the fire was not consuming it. As he drew close, he heard God, the one who had called him, say, "Do not come any closer.... Take off your sandals, for the place you are standing is holy ground" (Exo. 3:5). The Bible doesn't say, but we can be sure that he did what he was told!

What made this austere and harsh desert place holy? Two things: the Holy One was present there, and His presence made it holy. It was also holy because God had set this desolate place apart for a particular purpose. Here He called His servant Moses and set him apart to lead His people out of slavery and into the promised land. The ground was holy because of who was there and what He was doing in that place.

So what establishes sex as holy—a sacred gift—for God's people? First, sex is holy because God is present when a husband and wife share the gift of sex. And second, sex is holy because God designed the gift of sexual intimacy as a way for the husband and wife to create the oneness of marriage. This is a bit of a mystery, but sex makes two people one. How? God created and declared it to be so.

We learn more about the meaning of the word *holy* from the scriptures. The first is the idea that something is perfect, unmatched, and pure. At least twenty-five times, the prophet Isaiah mentions God as "the Holy One of Israel." Interestingly, Peter's description of Jesus declares, "We believe and know that you are the Holy One of God" (John 6:69).

Holiness also relates to something that God has purposely identified as holy. In the Old Testament, the Ark of the Covenant was such an object. It represented God's throne amid His people, and it was a symbol of His presence and power with them wherever it went. There are quite a few miracles chronicled in the Old Testament associated with the ark. For example, with the presence of the ark, the waters of the Jordan River parted so the tribes of Israel could cross on dry land. Later, we find the ark present when the walls of Jericho collapsed so that the Israelites could conquer the city (Joshua 3:14–17, 6:6–21).

What may seem curious to us today is that hidden in the special golden box representing God's presence were not riches and priceless gems, but three unlikely items: a jar of bread, a stick, and two stones. What were these peculiar keepsakes, and why did God want them in His ark?

The three items each had great significance. The *pot of manna* was a stinging reminder that, despite what God had provided for them, the Israelites had rejected God's provision. It was a sign that the Holy One was worthy of their trust. The *staff* reminded the Israelites that they had repeatedly rejected God's authority in the past. It was a symbol that the Holy One was and always will be the supreme authority (Phil. 2:10–11).

What about the *two stones*? The two stone tablets were a reminder of the Ten Commandments. *Goodseed Resources* wrote, "God had chosen the Israelites as His special people. For the Israelites to qualify for that distinction, God had demanded one thing. They must obey His Law, the Ten Commandments."[53] This portion of God's Word also speaks about God's holy design for marriage. Exodus 20:14 records, "You shall not commit adultery." In other words, marriage is a grand part of God's plan and gift to us all—a sacred gift to be safeguarded and protected.

Several passages highlight how the Israelites were to obey God and be His special people. Deuteronomy 7:6 says, "For you are a people holy to the LORD your God. The LORD your God has chosen you out of all the peoples on the face of the earth to be his people, his treasured possession." The same purpose also applies to the church. In 1 Peter 2:9, we are told, "But you are a chosen people, a royal priesthood, a holy nation, God's special possession, that you may declare the praises of him who called you out of darkness into his wonderful light."

Finally, *holy* means to stir praise, worship, and even fear in a believer. This is how Peter responded when Jesus miraculously filled the boat with fish. "When Simon Peter saw this, he fell at Jesus' knees and said, 'Go away from me, Lord; I am a sinful man!'" (Matt. 5:8). Peter was stirred to a sense of unworthiness. This is clearly how Moses felt when he lay prostrate on the hot sand at Mount Horeb (Exo. 3:5).

How does all this relate to sex and marriage? Each of these four definitions of *holiness* applies to sex between a husband and a wife. First, sex is holy because the Holy One of Israel created it before sin ever entered the human story. In the beginning, sex was uncorrupted and spiritually pure.

Sex is also sacred because God set it apart to be so. As we noted about the Ark of the Covenant, it was regarded with great wonder and respect. The mystery of oneness between a man and a woman in the sex act is to be given a similarly holy and high regard. This certainly does not fit with much of the current language or concepts such as "casual sex" or "hooking up." Sex is to be treated with the honor afforded that which is holy, just like the ark.

Further, sex is holy because God set it apart from the beginning of time for His particular purpose. It is the unique purpose of representing Christ and the church (Eph. 5:31–32). This is a great mystery that was revealed in Christ. The incredible truth is that the intimacy expressed in the sexual union between a husband and wife is the representation of the intimacy between the Savior and the church, referred to as the *bride of Christ*.

Finally, sex is holy because it can guide us into an authentic experience of worship. The burning bush filled Moses with the awe and majesty of God. Similarly, the real knowledge of oneness that God made marital sex to be can bring us to a place of adoration and praise for God. It can leave us trembling at the wonder and beauty and love of the Holy One who is so gracious.

It is imperative for you to know that sex is holy. Why? It provides for you a vision of what God has planned for you. You can make choices now to obey God and enjoy many advantages for a lifetime by waiting. There are numerous benefits of saving sex until marriage.

1. You can give the person you marry the gift no one else will ever have.
2. You can avoid the emotional trauma and depression of having sex with different people.
3. You can learn self-respect.
4. You will learn to depend on God and self-control.
5. You will not have the worries of pregnancy and disease.
6. More importantly, you will please and honor God.

DISCUSSION STARTERS

1. What is your understanding of sex as sacred according to the scriptures?
2. In your view, what is the significance of the three items contained within the Ark of the Covenant?
3. What difference does it make for you to know that sex is sacred?
4. Can you see a difference in the lives of couples who believe in the sacred nature of sex?

DAY 23
EMBRACE EVERY PERSON'S WORTH

We see in Jesus a powerful example of treating people with dignity and love. In Matthew 9:36, we hear, "When he saw the crowds, he had compassion on them, because they were harassed and helpless, like sheep without a shepherd." Do we see people with care, delight, and generosity? Or, do we view them with suspicion, fear, and fault? Each of us chooses how we will look at others.

For the sake of simplicity, let's assume there are basically two ways of living. On the one hand, there is an open, generous, and kind way to live for others. On the other side, there is a suspicious, self-centered, separated way, for us. Jesus demonstrated the first way of being. He showed a thoroughly consistent life of holding God and others in one thought at a time. He cared about the lives of others, and his greatest passion was compassion.

According to Martin Buber, a great Jewish scholar, human beings may adopt two attitudes toward the world. He wrote about this in a famous book published in 1923 called *I and Thou*. We will replace the word *Thou* with the word *You* from this point forward. The book describes the two ways as *I-You* or *I-It*. I-You is a relation of person-to-person, while I-It is a relation of person-to-object. In the I-You relationship, human beings are aware of one another as having a significant degree in common. In this case, we see the person as real. They have hopes and dreams just like us.

In the I-You relationship, human beings do not recognize one another "as consisting of specific, isolated qualities, but engage in a dialogue involving each other's whole being. In the I-It relationship, on the other hand, human beings perceive each other as consisting of specific, isolated qualities, and view themselves as part of a world which consists of things."[54] I-You is a relationship of mutuality and reciprocity, while I-It is a relationship of separateness and detachment.

C. Terry Warner writes about these two ways of being in his book *Bonds That Make Us Free*.[55] In short, the I-It way of being views the other person as an object. The adapted sample list below from his book will help you to clarify the two.

I-It	I-You
worried about yourself	interested in others
insecure	secure, peaceful
selfish	sharing
rigid	flexible
scarcity-minded	abundance-minded
sees others as rivals	sees others as friends
lonely	supportive
self-centered	other-centered
lust-driven	love-propelled

Let's use a real-life example to illustrate what we are talking about. Of course, the names have been changed to protect personal identities. Trace the increase and growth of William's change into a different, I-It kind of person. William is fifteen years old and a sophomore in high school. This year he has started to take notice of girls, especially Tracy. She is in his calculus class, and he finds himself not just thinking that she is attractive. His thoughts have escalated to a predictable daily pattern of sexual lust and obsession. He wants to stop doing the wrong thing, which is lusting after Tracy. He told his friend Jerry about his struggle, and Jerry said, "What's the problem? All guys do that!" He knew he needed better advice.

There is a way to escape our self-absorption. We can release ourselves from the I-It condition. It involves the critical act of making a choice by which we indirectly choose our way of being. The Bible calls it to sin—and most people today don't want to speak the word. Why? The implication is that the recognition of sin lays the responsibility on us to examine and change ourselves. Who wants to face up to the fact that they have themselves to thank for their present dilemma?

The struggle became so intense for William that he decided to visit his pastor. He had known him a couple of years, and he liked and trusted Mr. Norton. So he called and set up an appointment for Saturday morning. William shared his battle, and Mr. Norton listened a long time before speaking. Finally, he commented, "William, you are not alone in your struggle. It is a struggle known by all men. One thing has helped me, and it is looking at girls in a relationship context, not as an object. There is a lot more to girls than their physical features. It isn't likely that you will lust after your sister or your mom. You see them as real people with multiple dimensions. You see them like a sister, mother, believer, someone's daughter, and so on."

They talked for another thirty minutes. Pastor Norton offered him a few practical ideas about what to do next time he saw Tracy at school. He pondered his pastor's words considerably over the weekend. He started to look at Tracy and other girls with new eyes and felt for her from a new heart. The hold of lust was losing its grip.

Monday morning, he saw Tracy in calculus class. Immediately, he put the brakes on his old thoughts. He saw her as a real person, the way Martin Buber described as I-You, not I-It. In his mind, he was saying, *Don't simply see her physical attributes. She is so much more. She is a real person with others in her life who love her. Certainly, God cares for her! God, I pray for her to know you and the power of your love.* The more William started to see her in a relational context, the more he became himself. He was less the self-absorbed boy and more becoming a man of God!

The goal of embracing every person's worth can be grounded in the biblical concept of the Imago Dei. *Imago Dei* means "the image of God," and the first biblical reference is found in Genesis 1:27: "So God created mankind in his own image, in the image of God he created them; male and female he created them." Jesus quoted this text in Matthew 19:4, when He said, " ... at the beginning the Creator 'made them male and female.'"

For Christ, women have an intrinsic value the same as men. Women are fashioned in the image of God similarly as men are. Jesus viewed women as genuine persons. They weren't simple objects of male desire. It is a fact of considerable historical importance that Jesus elevated the status of women.

Sue Bohlin, a writer for Probe Ministries, quotes from Alvin Schmidt in his book *How Christianity Changed the World* these remarkable words:

> Jesus' treatment of women was very different from the culture. The low status that the Greek, Roman, and Jewish woman had for centuries was significantly affected by the appearance of Jesus Christ. His actions and teachings raised the status of women to new heights, often to the consternation and dismay of his friends and enemies. By word and deed, He went against the ancient, taken-for-granted beliefs and practices that defined a woman as socially, intellectually, and spiritually inferior.

> The humane and respectful way Jesus treated and responded to the Samaritan woman at the well (recorded in John 4) may not appear unusual to readers in today's Western culture. What He did was extremely rare, even radical. He ignored the anti-Samaritan prejudices along with the prevailing view that saw women as inferior beings.[56]

Jesus offered women status and respect equal to men. He broke with the antifemale culture of His era, and He set a standard for His followers. He set the countercultural direction for the New Testament Church.

DISCUSSION STARTERS

1. Do you perceive life more through the I-It or I-You lens?
2. What do you think is the meaning and significance of the Imago Dei concept found in Genesis 1:27?
3. What do you think Jesus says to teens (guys or girls) who lust and view porn?
4. How do you understand the practical implications of Jesus' life and message when it comes to how the sexes relate to each other?

DAY 24
PRACTICE A LIFE OF GRATITUDE

Mick Jagger penned all the lyrics to a particular well-known song except the line "Can't get no satisfaction." He and the Rolling Stones made this rock ballad famous. The lyrics deal with what Jagger saw as the two segments of America, the real and the counterfeit. He sang about a man looking for integrity and not being able to find it. Jagger experienced the vast commercialism of America in a big way on his tours. He later learned to capitalize on it as the Rolling Stones became wealthy through sponsorships and merchandising in the United States.

Today many find it difficult to find satisfaction due to the influence of advertising. Images of new products make the things you have appear out of style. The advertisers want you to think that you will be happier with their products. Pope John Paul II wrote, "Young people are threatened ... by the evil use of advertising techniques that stimulate the natural inclination to avoid hard work by promising the immediate satisfaction of every desire."[57]

Porn is the most dangerous promoter of anger, discontent, lust, and self-gratification in our culture today. It causes dissatisfaction cultivated by the airbrushed images and always willing "lovers." Porn creates discontentment toward

- real human bodies,
- sex reserved for marriage, and
- marital fulfillment.

This is not to say that all dissatisfaction is sinful. For instance, there is nothing wrong with anger at immorality and discrimination. We should be angry with these wrongs and work to resolve them.

The kind of dissatisfaction we are talking about here is the kind that says, "I want more things, more pleasure, more luxury in life—and I'm entitled to it. I'd better take over the responsibility for myself; God isn't doing a good enough job."

However, discontentment is not only an insult to God; it is also a way we rob ourselves of the joy we might have each day. God wants us to focus on what we have now instead of obsessing about what we might have in the future. Moreover, as we become restless, resentful, and bitter, other people naturally prefer not to be around us.

God intends for contentment to be a characteristic of every Christian life. However, not all teens enjoy peace. What about you? Are you influenced in an unhealthy way by the materialism and greed in our culture? Or do you have an attitude of complaining and ingratitude?

One of the best ways to combat discontentment and lust is through the practice of gratitude. Dissatisfaction is generally an attitude that questions the goodness, faithfulness, and provision of God in your life. Counselors widely agree that many teens are fixated on porn and masturbation as a way of escaping pain, compensating for disappointment, and avoiding difficult circumstances.

Contentment learns to cope with these things in the light of God's sufficiency and grace. Christian author Jerry Bridges wrote, "The contented person experiences the sufficiency of God's provision for his needs and the sufficiency of God's grace for his circumstances."[58] The apostle Paul shared what God had spoken to him: "My grace is sufficient for you, for my power is made perfect in weakness. Therefore, I will boast all the more gladly about my weaknesses, so that Christ's power may rest on me" (2 Cor. 12:9).

Gratitude is also a weapon against discontentment, lust for more, and wrongdoing. As Christians still living in our "flesh," as Paul calls it in Romans chapter 6 and 7, we fight sin daily. The practice of gratitude will always diminish the presence and power of lust. Gerald Good stated, "If you want to turn your life around, try thankfulness. It will change your life mightily."[59]

Romans 1 identifies the predicament of all people who do not have a renewing faith in God: "For although they knew God, they did not honor him as God or give thanks to him, but they became futile in their thinking, and their foolish hearts were darkened" (vs. 21).

In other words, we grow in understanding and wisdom by giving thanks and honor to God. Gratitude in the good times and bad times is a tool to do that. Paul says, "...give thanks in all circumstances; for this is God's will for you in Christ Jesus" (1 Thess. 5:18).

There are many ways to practice gratitude. It's not inappropriate to want things and to acquire them by healthy and lawful means. But wanting can quickly turn into coveting as we fixate on the stuff we want and ignore the good things that we have.

Covetousness is an excessive wish to have more than you already have. It is expressly forbidden in the Ten Commandments (see Exo. 20:17) and in the New Testament also (see Col. 3:5). Covetousness usually starts with discontentment, the disturbing thought that what you have isn't good enough.

Gratitude helps us to restore this relational problem. Gratitude helps us to process the many ways that God has supplied our needs and more. It helps us look to Him as the most precious gift we could ever know. Being thankful for His Word, our hope in Jesus for salvation, as well as the earthly good things that He has given us to enjoy, is an excellent place to start.

Here are some other ways to practice gratitude and loosen the grip of discontentment and lust.

- Tell God each day what you are thankful for in your prayers.
- Focus on what's right in your life more than what's wrong.

- When a friend or family member annoys you, remember why you love them.
- Every day tell God one thing you like about your body.
- Compare well—when you find yourself envying someone, focus on what you have that other people don't.

You can find satisfaction and contentment despite the influence of advertisers and pornographers. God is your faithful and abundant provider. He loves you and is working in every aspect of your life. You can live content, pure, and free. That is His plan and destiny for you.

DISCUSSION STARTERS

1. Do you think Mick Jagger's message is the last word: "Can't get no satisfaction?"
2. What kind of discontentment do you think is created by exposure to pornography?
3. Is discontentment a spiritual issue reflecting on your relationship with God?
4. Just how much difference can the practice of gratitude make in your life?

DAY 25
AN ENDURING TRUST IN GOD'S GRACE

The Bible tells us that if we fight and endure for a short time, the trial will pass and the temptation will fade away. We must be ever ready for battle and to face challenges. C. H. Spurgeon preached a sermon on May 11, 1916, that said, in part, "There is a warfare in which all of us are engaged. What is life but a great battle, lasting from our earliest days until we sheathe sword in death?"[60]

If we will submit ourselves to God and resist, the outcome is assured. James 4:7 states, "Submit yourselves, then, to God. Resist the devil, and he will flee from you." With this assurance in mind, here are some additional practical ways to face your temptations and trials. These are simple but powerful suggestions. You are encouraged to put them into practice.

First, learn the truth and uncover the lies. Temptations have a way of blinding us to what lies ahead in the future. They focus on a moment of pleasure, and they deliver a quick payoff. Yes, sin can be gratifying for a short time, but will it be worth it long term?

Second, search the Word of God and wait on Him. Ask yourself, *What does God's Word say about this situation or choice?* If you are patient, He will provide the needed guidance and help. The psalmist proclaimed, "I wait for the LORD, my whole being waits, and in his word I put my hope" (Ps. 130:5).

Third, examine and hold on to the great promises of God. God has a great purpose for your life. It is wise to recognize God's good intentions and to be receptive to His wisdom and knowledge. Consider these words of the psalmist: "The fear of the LORD is the beginning of wisdom; all who follow his precepts have good understanding. To him belongs eternal praise" (Ps. 111:10).

Fourth, look for God's help, and He will provide a way out. You don't have to give in or go back to a life of bondage. You don't have to live in guilt and shame. Remember, as a Christian, you are not in the battle alone. His grace will be enough to help you overcome every temptation.

David Erik Jones was trapped in sexual addiction for over twenty years. It all started in his teen years when he was drawn into pornography and held captive by its lustful grip. Today, he shares his story of how God provided him a way out. In his book *My Struggle, Your Struggle*, he speaks about the available victory. He writes, "I want to encourage you to take His hand. Let His word be a lamp unto your feet. He will light the way and show you what to do. Then take steps of faith, follow what you know to be true, commit yourself to obey whatever truth God reveals to your heart. If you will trust Him, and make an effort, He will draw closer than you could ever imagine. He will transform your life and bless you incredibly."[61]

Paul wrote, "Forgetting what is behind and straining toward what is ahead, I press on toward the goal to win the prize for which God has called me heavenward in Christ Jesus" (Phil. 3:12–14). The language he uses is that of the athletic field of competition. He encourages us to forget what lies behind. What does that mean?

It means that we can live differently than the rest of the world. There is no way we will ever be without sin. We can, however, live a pure life through Christ and with the supernatural power of the Holy Spirit. Paul says, "Therefore, if anyone is in Christ, he is a new creation: The old has gone, the new has come!" (2 Cor. 5:17). We are changed, and we are in the ongoing process of change—becoming more and more like Christ.

This happens when we allow God to replace the self as our

master. When we let the Spirit guide us, warn us, comfort us, and protect us, then we are not bound by the self or self-gratification. As Paul describes, "I have been crucified with Christ and I no longer live, but Christ lives in me. The life I now live in the body, I live by faith in the Son of God, who loved me and gave himself for me" (Gal. 2:20).

This humbling of the self is always present in the life of someone who is pressing on and becoming more like Christ. We can never be pure without humility because humility is how we give up self-rule in favor of the One who is sovereign—God. Humility is the attitude of, "I can't do any of this on my own. I need God. There must be more of Him and less of me. Lord, help me to get out of the way."

This attitude leads to purity. Can you see how? Humility raises Christ to the center of your life. When this happens, your happiness and pleasure take a back seat to God. You make decisions instead based on what pleases and honors Him.

When you slip up, you confess it and continue a process of self-examination. Your goal in this situation is to press on to learn from your sin and grow. The practice of self-examination and confession is an ancient one—and much needed today. The first-century Roman philosopher Seneca said, "We should every night call ourselves to an account; what infirmities have I mastered today? What passions opposed? What temptation resisted? What virtues acquired?"[62]

There is much to be gained from this examination and reflection. The humble of heart seek in all their ways to come under the direction of Jesus Christ and become more like Him. The following process will add to a transformation of your life: (1) set aside a specific time for this purpose, (2) select a space with limited distractions, and (3) determine a set of questions to help examine your life with Jesus Christ.

The list that follows is an excellent place to begin. Here are some examples for you to consider for a weekly pure heart examination.

- Did I have quality time with God through prayer and reading the Word?
- Did I spend adequate, quality time in worship and fellowship with other believers?
- Am I utilizing and maintaining my accountability relationships?
- Did I exercise my body sufficiently for good health?
- Did I practice self-control with second looks, lust, and objectifying of people?
- Did I implement my action plan in times of temptation?
- Did I spend a healthy amount of time with friends and family?
- Am I working in some way toward my dream goals or destiny?

When you have done this for a while, you will find your rhythm and method. You may cover all the points each day or dwell more on one than another. This prayerful reflection will produce a tremendous spiritual benefit.

Paul encourages us by saying, "Forgetting what is behind" (Phil. 3:13). In this grand adventure, we live by a new faith that overcomes fear, dread, and uncertainty. Fear is the voice that says you can't make it. Dread lies and tells you there is no promise for tomorrow. Doubt is the denial of God's power and work.

We are drawn and empowered by a great grace that overcomes failure. Don't give up! Press on! We live called to "throw off everything that hinders and the sin that so easily entangles. And let us run with perseverance the race marked out for us, fixing our eyes on Jesus, the pioneer and perfecter of faith. For the joy set before him, he endured the cross, scorning its shame, and sat down at the right hand of the throne of God" (Heb. 12:1–2). Keep your eyes on the One who has already won and assured you of the victory. Keep your eyes on Him. Even if you stumble, He will carry you.

The 1992 Olympic Games were convened in Barcelona, Spain, and the runner most people thought would win the four-hundred-meter run was Derek Redmond of England. Only 150 meters out, his Achilles tendon snapped. A startled gasp burst from the crowd as they watched him stumble, then catch himself and begin to hobble. In excruciating pain, he limped down the course, remaining determined to cross the finish line, no matter how long it took. Other runners sped by as a solitary figure pushed his way out of the stands and onto the track. The man put his son's arm over his shoulder and helped him to finish the race. It was Redmond's father!

This was a marvelous picture of what God's enormous mercy and grace are like when failure or brokenness hinders us from achieving our goals. Like Derek Redmond, we need to press on. If we stay on the track, we can go the distance because we have a Heavenly Father who will come to us, put His arms around us, uphold us, and see us through to the end.

The Lord is calling each of us to go the distance. Paul expressed that calling by writing, "I press on toward the goal to win the prize for which God has called me heavenward in Christ Jesus" (Phil. 3:14). He promises to be with us each step.

DISCUSSION STARTERS

1. What do you think of the four practical ways to handle temptations and trials? Which one works best for you?
2. Do you share the optimism and faith of Pastor David Erik Jones?
3. Will you humbly implement the practice of self-examination as discussed in this daily reading?
4. What does the story of Derek Redmond and his dad in the 1992 Olympic Games tell you about the beauty and character of God?

DAY 26

PURITY IS ABOUT PLEASING GOD

When it comes to the opposite sex, love can be very confusing and tempting. Do you love them? Do they love you? Whether you are dating or not, your purity will be tested. Having a sense of what to make of your life and dating is an important thing. If you have a vision for your life, it will be all the better.

The most asked question in relationships is, "How far is too far?" There are two likely reasons you might ask that question. The first is you don't want to sin, and you want to know the rules to keep yourself pure in God's eyes. The second is you want to enjoy yourself and go as far as possible without the guilt. Hayley and Michael DiMarco write, "All of us have a choice to make in relation to others: we can love them for our pleasure, their pleasure, or for God's pleasure."[63]

As is true in most areas of our lives, we are concerned about our physical well-being. The scriptures repeatedly remind us that purity is directed to God's pleasure, and this includes the use of our bodies. We are advised in 1 Corinthians 10:31, "Whether you eat or drink or whatever you do, do all to the glory of God." You can see this truth in 1 Corinthians 6:20: "You were bought with a price. So, glorify God in your body." God did not intend for the body to be used for impure purposes.

Purity is really about the condition of your heart and its devotion. It is not a list of things you can do and cannot do, such as you can hold hands, kiss on the lips, and hug so long as your hand is above the waist. Of course, physical boundaries are essential. The person who is dedicated to the honor and pleasure of God above all will know what to do. God gives guidance and wisdom to those who ask, so it is a good idea to ask Him for help in setting your physical boundaries during dating.

If you genuinely think about honoring God and the future of the person you are dating, you will steer clear of putting yourself in a compromising situation. Where do you draw the line? How far are you willing to go sexually before marriage? What is right for you, and how do you maintain your decision?

You can do two things to help prepare. First, set a firm limit on where you will stop the physical contact. Decide now. This is far wiser than waiting until the heat is up and then trying to decide. Be conservative about where to draw the line. Sexual activity can escalate quickly in the passion of the moment. Next, take this decision to the Lord in prayer. Ask Him if He is pleased with where you have decided to draw the line. If you have any doubt, then go back to the Lord in prayer and ask Him to guide you.

Remember that God's standard is quite explicit. Paul writes, "Among you there must not be even a hint of sexual immorality, or any kind of impurity.... These are improper for God's holy people" (Eph. 5:13). So it is best to draw the line in a safe place, not leading us into temptation. Jesus even taught us to pray as a priority focus: "And lead us not into temptation, but deliver us from the evil one" (Matt. 6:13).

Where will you draw the line? This is a good question for you to think about and pray for God's guidance. It will be helpful to you in your dating relationships in the days ahead. More importantly, you must never forget that purity is walking in the love of Father God revealed in Jesus Christ.

Purity is not about a fixed point on a line that you cross or don't cross. It is first and foremost about a relationship with Christ and your desire to follow Him. There will be moments of great victory.

There will be times of sadness and letdown. It is all a part of the process of growing up. There is a way for you to make the right choice that turns temptation into purity. You can succeed in doing this by embracing three truths:

1. You were not born pure. You were born into a sinful world that is at war. God wants to give you a fulfilling life, but there is an enemy who wants to steal it from you and destroy you. The world is fundamentally broken and cannot find peace apart from God and obedience to His perfect will.

2. You will face temptation—including the monster of lust—many times in your life, but the ordinary look or thought is not a sin. It is an opportunity to develop purity by pursuing Christ and making the right choices, with His help.

3. You can become pure. There is nothing that says you must sin. It is imperative that you believe this truth because there is a power that overcomes—the power of Jesus' suffering, death, and resurrection. This is made a reality through the indwelling of the Holy Spirit.

The gifts of your mind, your body, your relationships, and sex are to be directed to Christ. Your motivation for purity must be based on what Christ has done for you, or it's not really purity but a cheap imitation. The love of Christ for us cost Him everything—and He paid the price gladly! God gave you gifts so you could use them to point others to Christ—to His beauty, His glory, and His majesty. You can't do that by engaging in sexual relations outside of marriage (Eph. 5:3).

You were given life not to use as you please but to give back to God. God longs to fill you with His Spirit. God gave you the gift of self so that you will yield it entirely to Him. The clean life is 100 percent free from self (that is, self-gratification). The genuine person is radically dedicated to one thing: the glory and honor of God.

Ultimately, all our trouble comes down to self-gratification. This happens when you think or say, "I deserve it" or "I am entitled." It comes when you look for things that bring you pleasure and thereby reason you can have whatever you want. When you base your life on comfort, ease, or happiness, you make life self-serving, not about serving God. Andrew Murray put it this way: "Every time you please yourself, you deny Jesus. It is one of the two. You must please Him only and deny self. Or you must please yourself and deny Him."[64]

DISCUSSION STARTERS

1. In 1 Corinthians 10:31, the Bible says, "Whether you eat or drink or whatever you do, do all to the glory of God." What does this verse communicate to you?

2. Do you agree that "purity is really about the condition of your heart and its devotion"?

3. What do you think of the statement that "there is a power that overcomes—the power of Jesus' suffering, death, and resurrection. This is made a reality through the indwelling of the Holy Spirit"?

4. What do you think of the statement by Andrew Murray in today's reading?

DAY 27

BEGINNING WITH THE END IN MIND

Beginning with the end in mind can be a big help in getting a clearer picture of what you want to do with your life. You most likely don't have a complete picture of that goal. However, you can start to think beyond today and think about the path you want to take toward your future.

A lawyer approached Jesus and asked, "What must I do to inherit eternal life?" (Luke 10:26). Jesus replied, "'Love the Lord your God with all your heart and with all your soul and with all your strength and with all your mind'; and, 'Love your neighbor as yourself'" (Luke 10:27). Jesus taught the message that life is about relationships, starting with a passionate love for God and learning to love your neighbor as yourself.

Not having an end in mind can be a huge problem. You may recall the funny conversation in Lewis Carroll's *Alice's Adventures in Wonderland:*

> "Would you tell me please which way I ought to go from here?"
> "That depends a good deal on where you want to get to," said the Cat.
> "I don't much care where—" said Alice.
> "Then it doesn't matter which way you go," said the Cat.[65]

It is much better to have some sense of direction because it offers some motivation. We find it hard to move on without some incentive. If we know why we are doing something, then it is easier to give our best efforts.

If we don't decide the direction for our lives, we have an enemy who will try to seduce us to take a path of destruction. Jesus described the Enemy as one who has plans "to kill, steal, and destroy" (John 10:10). We best understand the direction of our lives by knowing Jesus. He said, "I am the way and the truth and the life. No one comes to the Father except through me" (John 14:6).

Understanding the end is crucial in maintaining a proper perspective—both for the foolish and the wise. Without understanding our purpose, it is all too easy to become discouraged and distracted. Perhaps this is the reason Paul states, "And let us not be weary in well doing: for in due season we shall reap, if we faint not" (Gal. 6:9). Losing sight of our goal can cause us to become weary and quit.

When we lose sight of what life is all about, we are prone to get pulled into the world's understanding of success. We begin thinking that our worth is determined by material things, by power, or by fame. Then, as we start to derive our sense of value from these things, we miss the mark of our real identity and destiny as children of God.

When we do what Stephen R. Covey calls "begin with the end in mind," we can make better decisions.[66] Let's say that you want to grow in your love for the Lord. That is certainly a noble and worthy goal. Here are five ways to begin with the end in mind:

1. **Start at the base of the cross.** The cross is the beginning of our experience with God, not the end. Encourage your heart by embracing the fullness of Christ's forgiveness! Take courage and live with the glad assurance, "There is no fear in love. But perfect love drives out fear, because fear has to do with punishment. The one who fears is not made perfect in love" (1 John 4:18).

2. **Remember that God couldn't love you any more than He already does.** Christ's sacrifice covers all our sins with no exception. There are at least eighteen times in the Bible when we are described in some way or another as His bride. This means that He looks upon us with the same passion and eagerness as the bridegroom does his bride on their wedding day. Try this: the next time you go to a wedding, observe as the bride comes down the aisle, and then also glance back to the groom. Then, remember that is what the Lord feels for you every second of your life!

3. **Above all, heed the voice of God.** The Enemy is known as "the accuser of the brethren" (Rev. 12:10). The very term *devil* means "slanderer." Satan cannot read our minds, but he can put thoughts into our minds. In 2 Corinthians 10:5, we read, "We are taking every thought captive according to the obedience of Christ." So what sort of thoughts are we to take captive? Well, some thoughts come to your mind that are not in agreement with what God says about you. Ideas also enter your thinking that are contrary to what God reveals about Himself.

   God desires that we have confidence in His Word more than we trust our feelings, more than we believe how things appear. God's Word is more reliable than anything we may think. David, in the Psalms, said, "Your Word ... is a light to my path" (Ps. 119:105). St. Augustine stated with delight, *"God loves each of us as if there were only one of us."*[67]

4. **Nurture your love.** You may love someone very much. Growing your love with God, or nurturing that love, is accomplished in much the same way. There are specific actions you take to keep the passion alive. You talk to Him through prayer, thanksgiving, and singing. You listen to Him often through His Word, but not hurriedly or superficially. You'll spend time in the morning reading just a few verses, meditating on them, and seeking the help

of the Holy Spirit to live by the living Word. In our overly busy culture, this gives us time to hear, understand, and honor Him.

5. **The practice of praise**. You may be a closet Eeyore, meaning a positive attitude does not come naturally for you. However, you know that there are habits that nurture praise—singing, humming, and thanking God throughout the day. Why? Because they focus us on the truth of who He is, not the misleading notions suggested by circumstances. Moreover, you know that how you feel doesn't affect whether or not you praise Him. Paul, who endured considerable pain and disappointment, wrote, "Rejoice always. Pray without ceasing. In everything give thanks, for this is the will of God in Christ Jesus concerning you" (1 Thess. 5:16–18). That's God's will for us.

Let's say that you want to grow in your love for your neighbor. That is a high end to keep in mind. Here are five ways to do that:

1. TRY TO SEE YOUR NEIGHBOR THROUGH THE EYES OF JESUS

Love your neighbors, whoever they are, by seeing them through the eyes of Jesus. You can look past the obvious, the outer shells, and into their eyes, their hearts, and their circumstances. If you are blinded by your bitterness or anger, ask Jesus to give you His eyes to see others as He does.

2. ASK FOR FORGIVENESS AND OFFER IT

Yes, you can ask for forgiveness for the strongholds within your own heart that keep you from understanding or loving another. If you are closed off to or indifferent toward a person, confess it before the Lord and ask for His forgiveness. If you need to ask for forgiveness from your neighbor, you can humble yourself and apologize. If you need to extend mercy toward a person, you can offer it.

3. PRAY FOR OTHERS

You love your neighbors by praying for them—even if it's through gritted teeth at first. You ask God to give you a new heart, and you ask with faith in His provision. You can pray for your neighbors' circumstances, salvation, and walk with the Lord.

4. REJOICE AND MOURN WITH THEM

We can walk alongside our neighbors. Paul stated, "Rejoice with those who rejoice; mourn with those who mourn" (Rom. 12:15). We can attune our spirits with theirs as we say, "I'll give thanks with you, and I'll cry with you." We'll bear the burden of their pain and anguish because we know that Christ is the ultimate burden-bearer.

5. BE TEACHABLE AND HUMBLE

Christ's ways are often difficult and challenging, and we'll choose the harder path. We'll be teachable, and we'll learn. We'll allow our neighbors to challenge our hearts without taking offense or becoming bitter. We'll accept constructive criticism as the pathway that draws us closer to Christ. We won't be self-righteous or act like a know-it-all.

Make your life extraordinary. Howard Thurman once said, "Don't ask yourself what the world needs. Ask yourself what makes you come alive and go do that because what the world needs is people who have come alive."[68] If you want to "come alive," there is no better way than to keep the end in mind of loving God with your whole being and learning to love others!

DISCUSSION STARTERS

1. What does it mean to you to "begin with the end in mind"?
2. What are you willing to do to grow in your love for God?
3. What are you willing to do to grow in your love for others?
4. Since reading this book, have you heard from God about the "end in mind" regarding the gift of your sexuality?

DAY 28
IT'S TIME FOR REVIVAL!

Things may never have been this bad in all our history in the United States of America. There has been a massive moral decline, soaring divorce rates, and alarming crime rates. The fabric of our society has unraveled, and it is hard to find basic respect and decency. We could use revival!

You have most likely heard the word *revival*. Some churches publicize that they will have a revival, with the dates, times, and names of speakers. In truth, if it is a bona fide revival, then it is not something churches can start or stop but something God supernaturally achieves. When this happens, God's people come back to life again.

The word *revive* means to restore something to its original condition. It is something similar to people who like to restore old furniture. They will take an old piece of furniture and then work to make it look like it did in its original condition. It involves many different steps:

1. Apply stripper and scrape off the finish.
2. Brush off the remaining finish.
3. Sand it thoroughly.
4. Apply primer.
5. Sand smooth and apply new finish.
6. Add another layer of color and detail.
7. Apply a final clear finish.

Similarly, to be revived means to return to God's original design. Revival is more than just an emotional experience. It is essentially the beginning of a new love for and obedience to God. Whenever this resurgence happens, there is repentance in the hearts of people and a change in the relationships between them.

I like the way Jeremiah describes it: "Thus says the Lord: 'Stand in the ways and see, and ask for the old paths, where the good way is, and walk in it; Then you will find rest for your souls. But they said, 'We will not walk in it'" (Jer. 6:16 NKJV). We don't need anything new. There is a crying need to go back to the very standards God has provided us, and we need to live by them.

Repentance means a willingness to change. Repentance says, "I am sorry, and I will stop what I am doing." The Bible declares, "Godly sorrow brings repentance that leads to salvation and leaves no regret" (2 Cor. 7:10).

God provides a remedy for the healing of our nation, and it includes repentance. He declares, "If my people, who are called by my name, will humble themselves and pray and seek my face and turn from their wicked ways, then I will hear from heaven, and I will forgive their sin and will heal their land" (2 Chron. 7:14). God has kindly provided a way for us to be forgiven and healed. We need to humble ourselves, pray, and turn away from our wicked ways.

We need a revival in the church, but it must first start with us individually. Ask yourself: Am I personally revived? Gypsy Smith, a nineteenth-century revivalist, used to stand, draw a circle around his feet, and then say, "Lord, please send revival, and start inside this circle."[69] Inevitably, revival begins with us.

You may be saying, "But I am only a teen. How can I possibly make a difference?" God has been faithful in every generation to bring revival to His people. These movements have often been very evident among young people. As we will see in the following stories, history tells the role of young people in the revivals.

In the Old Testament, there is the account of Joshua and the generation under twenty. Deuteronomy records, "And the little ones that you said would be taken captive, your children who do not yet know good from bad—they will enter the land. I will give it to them and they will take possession of it" (1:39).

Here are a couple of additional Old Testament revivals. Josiah, the king who was a boy, started a resurgence. "In the eighth year of his reign, while he was still young, he began to seek the God of his father, David. In his twelfth year, he began to purge Judah and Jerusalem of high places, Asherah poles and idols" (2 Chron. 34:3). What about Jeremiah, the young prophet? Jeremiah 1:6-7 says, "'Alas, Sovereign LORD,' I said, 'I do not know how to speak; I am too young.' But the LORD said to me, 'Do not say, 'I am too young.' You must go to everyone I send you to and say whatever I command you.'"

In the New Testament, John the Baptist was likely in his twenties when he began his public ministry. Mark says, "Now John was clothed with camel's hair and with a leather belt ... and he ate locusts and wild honey" (1:16). Most folks don't know, but John's moral influence lived on significantly for several hundred years. Who says that a young person can't have an impact on history?

God wants to bring a revival to our lives and our country. It needs to begin with us as individuals. Do you want renewal in your spiritual life? God is ready and willing to bring it about through the power of His Holy Spirit. What we are talking about here is of far greater importance than reviving and restoring furniture. Here are some recommendations adapted from Bill Bright that will help bring that revival and refreshing to your heart.

- Love God with all your heart, soul, and mind (Deut. 6:5).
- Ask the Holy Spirit to reveal any unconfessed sin in your life.
- If you have hurt someone, ask for their forgiveness.
- Ask the Lord to search and purify your heart daily.
- Ask the Holy Spirit to guard your walk against complacency and mediocrity.

- Praise and give thanks to God daily in all ways, regardless of your circumstances.
- Refuse to obey the desires of the flesh (Gal. 5:16,17).
- Surrender your life to Jesus Christ as your Savior and Lord. Develop utter dependence on Him with total submission and humility.
- Study the attributes of God.
- Hunger and thirst after righteousness (Matt. 5:6).
- Appropriate the continual fullness and control of the Holy Spirit by faith in God's command (Eph. 5:18) and promise (1 John 5:14,15).
- Read, study, meditate on, and memorize God's holy Word daily (Col. 3:16).
- Pray without ceasing (1 Thess. 5:17).
- Endeavor to share Christ daily in your life.[70]

Will you pray for a great revival among teens and young people to love and serve the Lord? What a joy it would be if young Christians today responded to God in radical obedience and service. Let us be like David, who "served the purpose of God in his generation."

DISCUSSION STARTERS

1. What do you think Paul means when he says, "Godly sorrow brings repentance that leads to salvation and leaves no regret" (2 Cor. 7:10)?
2. What biblical evidence do you know about young people who played a role in revival?
3. What might bring revival and refreshing to your spirit?
4. What gifts and abilities might God use in you to change the lives of others?

NOTES

1   Bonnie Rochman, "The Results Are In: First National Study of Teen Masturbation," Time, August 11, 2011, http://healthland.time.com/2011/08/11/boys-masturbate-more-than-girls-seriously/.

2   *Merriam-Webster*, s.v. "masturbation," https://www.merriam-webster.com/dictionary/masturbation.

3   Tim Kimmel, "Sex, Kids, and the Big Discussion," 09/01/2009, http://family matters.net/blog/2009/09/01/sex-kids-and-the-big-discussion/.

4   James Dobson, 1989. 83–84. Cited in Mark Regnerus, *Forbidden Fruit: Sex & Religion in the Lives of American Teenagers* (Oxford: Oxford UP, 2007), 262.

5   Joe McIlhaney and Freda Bush. *Hooked: New Science on How Casual Sex Is Affecting Our Children* (Chicago: Northfield Publishing, 2008), 21.

6   Joe Carter, " Things You Should Know about Pornography and the Brain," May 8, 2013, http://www.thegospelcoalition.org/article/9-things-you-should-know-about-pornography-and-the-brain.

7   Nancy Andreasen. *Brave New World* (New York: Oxford University Press, 2001).

8   Joelle Chase, "Irenaeus: Reminding Us Who We Are," June 28, 2012, https://spectrummagazine.org/article/joelle-chase/2012/06/28/irenaeus-reminding-us-who-we-are.

9   Personal Letter from Lewis to Keith Masson found in the Collected Letters of C. S. Lewis, Volume 3.

10 Ron Rolheiser, "God's Pleasure in Our Action," February 23, 2015, http://ronrolheiser.com/gods-pleasure-in-our-action/#.XBuIaFxKiUk.

11 Diane Howard, "On Wings of Eagles: The Sequel to Chariots of Fire," Sonoma Christian Home, November 2, 2017, retrieved May

28, 2019, https://sonomachristianhome.com/2017/11/on-wings-of-eagles-the-sequel-to-chariots-of-fire/.

12   John Piper. *The Dangerous Duty Delight: The Glorified God and the Satisfied Soul* (Colorado Springs: Multnomah, 2001), 55.

13   Quotes, retrieved April 29, 2019, https://www.quotes.net/quote/19669.

14   Focus on the Family. The Porn Phenomenon, retrieved May 6, 2019, https://www.focusonthefamily.com/socialissues/citizen-magazine/the-porn-phenomenon.

15   Dannah Gresh. *What Are You Waiting For?* (Colorado Springs: Waterbrook Press, 2011), 78.

16   Lydia Sweatt, "13 Quotes About Making Life Choices," October 6, 2006, https://www.success.com/13-quotes-about-making-life-choices/.

17   Letter published in *Memoir and Remains of the Rev. Robert Murray McCheyne* (Edinburgh, 1894) 293.

18   National Fatherhood Initiative, "The Proof Is In: Father Absence Harms Children," U.S. Census Bureau 2017, https://www.fatherhood.org/father-absence-statistic.

19   Tim Gardner. *Sacred Sex* (Colorado Springs: Waterbrook Press, 2002), 8.

20   Brennan Manning. *Ruthless Trust: The Ragamuffin's Path to God* (San Francisco: HarperCollins, 2002), 19.

21   Robert Poole, "Looting Irag," Smithsonian Magazine, February, 2008, https://www.smithsonianmag.com/arts-culture/looting-iraq-16813540/#t7B0bu79e8c5fHOU.99.

22   SSNET Web Team, "Christian Sexuality," January 25, 1998, http://ssnet.org/ qrtrly/eng/98a/less06.html.

23   Joe Ricchuiti, "God's Design for Sexuality," May 19, 2013, https://delriobiblechurch.com/online-sermons/577/.

24   Brennan Manning. *The Ragamuffin Gospel: Good News for the Bedraggled, Beat-Up, and Burnt Out* (Colorado Springs: Multnomah Publishing, 2005).

25   Douglas Weiss. *Clean: Proven Strategies for Men Committed to Sexual Integrity* (New York: Thomas Nelson, 2013), 128.

26   Christian Quotes. "101 Quotes from Jeremy Taylor," retrieved May 6, 2019, https://www.christianquotes.info/quotes-by-author/jeremy-taylor-quotes/#axzz5aWrMrS6g.

27   Barnabus Piper, "The 50 Best Quotes from the Ragamuffin Gospel," August 21, 2018, https://theblazingcenter.com/2018/08/ragamuffin-gospel.html.

28   Nick Vujicic. *Life Without Limits: Inspiration for a Ridiculously Good Life* (Colorado Springs: Waterbrook Press, 2010), 130.

29   Goodreads, retrieved July 17, 2019, https://www.goodreads.com/author/ quotes/3395320.Nick_Vujicic.

30   Lisa Jacks, "Rick Warren Quotes on Hope," April 3, 2015, https://www.newsmax.com/FastFeatures/rick-warren-quotes-hope-christian-evangelist/2015/05/03/ id/641828/.

31   Tyler Braun, "God Saves Us to Change Us," retrieved June 20, 2019, http://manofdepravity.com/2012/07/god-saves-us-to-change-us/.

32   James Bradley. *Flags of Our Father* (New York: Bantam Books, 2006), 174–175.

33   McChesney, Chris, Covey, Sean & Huling, Jim. *The Four Disciplines of Execution* (New York: Free Press, 2012).

34   Shay G. Meurer, "How to Increase the Odds of Reaching Your Goals," January 8, 2015, https://uponly.co/2015/01/08/how-to-increase-the-odds-of-reaching-your-goals-by-85-2/.

35   Harry Schaumburg. *False Intimacy: Understanding the Struggle of Sexual Addiction* (Colorado Springs: NavPress, 1997).

36   C.S. Lewis. *Mere Christianity* (New York: Simon and Schuster Touchstone edition, 1996), 109, 111.

37   Thomas Tarrant, "Pride and Humility", Winter 2011, http://www.cslewisinstitute.org/Pride_and_Humility_Page5.

38   Tim Sherfy, "Created for Greatness," October 31, 2011, https://www.evenifiwalkalone.com/2011/10/created-for-greatness/.

39   Steven Furtick. *Crash the Chatterbox.* (Colorado Springs: Multnomah Books, 2014), 39.

40   Steven Furtick. *Crash the Chatterbox.* (Colorado Springs: Multnomah Books, 2014), 46.

41   Daniel Henderson. *Think Before You Look: Avoiding the Consequences of Secret Temptation* (Chattanooga, TN: Living Ink Books, 2005), 64.

42   Mischel, W., Shoda, Y. & Rodriguez, M., L. (1989). Delay of gratification in children. *Science, 244*(4907), 933–937.

43   Ibid.

44   Ashley Fern, "Why Discipline Is So Essential to Your Character," June 14, 2013, https://www.elitedaily.com/why-discipline-is-so-important.

45   Stan Burman, "Quotes by Billy Graham on the Importance of Character," May 9, 2016, https://usefulquotations.wordpress.com/2016/05/09/quote-by-billy-graham-on-the-importance-of-character/.

46   Tim Gardner. *Sacred Sex: A Spiritual Celebration of Oneness in Marriage.* (Colorado Springs: Waterbrook Press: 2002), 21.

47 Travis Loeslie, "On the Freedom of a Christian," March 20, 2016, https://lutheranreformation.org/theology/on-the-freedom-of-a-christian/.

48 John Eldredge. *Waking the Dead: The Glory of a Heart Fully Alive* (Nashville, TN: Thomas Nelson Publishers, 2003), 13.

49 Brannan Manning. *Ruthless Trust: The Ragamuffin's Path to God* (New York: Harper Collins, 2002).

50 Brennan Manning. *The Ragamuffin Gospel: Good News for the Bedraggled, Beat-Up, and Burnt Out.* (Colorado Springs: Multnomah Books, 2005).

51 Brennan Manning. *Abba's Child: The Cry of the Heart for Intimate Belonging* (Colorado Springs: NavPress, 2002), 23.

52 Ibid., 64

53 Goodseed, "The Gate," retrieved May 29, 2019, https://www.goodseed.com/ark-of-the-covenant.html.

54 Audio Enlightenment, retrieved on June 1, 2019, http://www.audioenlightenment.com/i-and-thou-audio-sample.

55 C. Terry Warner. *Bonds That Make Us Free: Healing Our Relationships, Coming to Ourselves* (Salt Lake City: The Arbinger Institute, 2001).

56 Alvin Schmidt. *How Christianity Changed the World* (Grand Rapids, MI: Zondervan, 2001).

57 AZ Quotes, retrieved on May 15, 2019, https://www. azquotes. com/quote/ 226769.

58 Brainy Quotes, retrieved on May 10, 2019, https://gracequotes.org/topic/contentment/.

59 Goodreads, retrieved on May 17, 2019, https://www.goodreads.com/quotes/ 666437-if-you-want-to-turn-your-life-around-try-thankfulness.

60 C. H. Spurgeon, "The Battle of Life," www.spurgeon.org/sermons/3511.htm. Retrieved on 12/26/2018.

61 David Erik Jones. *My Struggle, Your Struggle: Breaking Free from Habitual Sin* (Maitland, FL: Xulon Press, 2007), 210.

62 Goodreads, "Seneca Quotes," retrieved on July 3, 2019, https://www.goodreads. com/quotes/207438-we-should-every-night-call-ourselves-to-an-account-what.

63 Hayley DiMarco and Michael DiMarco. *True Purity: More Than Just Saying "No" to You-Know-What* (Grand Rapids, MI: Revell, 2013), 42.

64 Goodreads, "Andrew Murray Quotes," retrieved on July 6, 2019, https://www.goodreads.com/author/quotes/13326.Andrew_Murray?page=14.

65 Lewis Carroll. *Alice's Adventures in Wonderland* (Sweden: Wisehouse Classics, 2017).

66   Sean Covey. *The 7 Habits of Highly Successful Teens* (New York: Simon & Schuster, 1998).

67   Brainy Quotes, "Saint Augustine Quotes," retrieved on May 15, 2019, https://www.brainyquote.com/quotes/saint_augustine_105351.

68   Murray, Andrew. *The Master's Indwelling*, available online at the Christian Classics Ethereal Library, http://www.ccel.org/ccel/murray/indwelling.html.

69   Nancy Leigh DeMoss, "Inside This Circle," February 18, 2014, https://www. reviveourhearts.com/podcast/seeking-him/inside-this-circle.

70   Bill Bright, "How to Have Personal Revival," Crosswalk.com, April 3, 2002, https://www.crosswalk.com/1130396/.

PURE TEENS: HONORING GOD, RELATIONSHIPS, AND SEX

War has been declared, and every teen needs a plan of action for living pure in this epic battlefield. *Pure Teens: Honoring God, Relationships, and Sex* is a valuable, practical resource for every Christian teen about relationships and sex—and why it is such a big deal to God. Not one to shy away from edgy topics, John candidly shares:

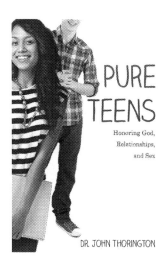

PURE
TEENS

Honoring God,
Relationships,
and Sex

DR. JOHN THORINGTON

- the ground-breaking science that explains the addictive power of cybersex
- straight talk about masturbation and pornography
- a battle plan for living porn free with sexual integrity
- a positive perspective about sacred sex
- the keys to a lifetime of fulfilling intimacy
- how to live boldly while honoring God

Each of the chapters in *Pure Teens* will help teens figure out God's roadmap in making decisions about how to honor Him, relationships, and sex.

This book is available at Amazon.com, Barnes and Noble, Focus on the Family.com, or www.restoringheartscounseling.com.

CALLING TEENS TO A LIFE OF FREEDOM, LOVE, AND GREATNESS IN CHRIST

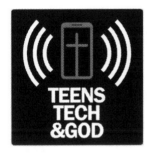

A podcast dedicated to equipping parents with the tools and knowledge to raise kids committed to God's purpose for sexuality, the family, and the honorable use of all technology.

with Dr. John Thorington
Find us on Apple Podcasts or go to
Drjohn.libsyn.com

www.restoringheartscounseling.com

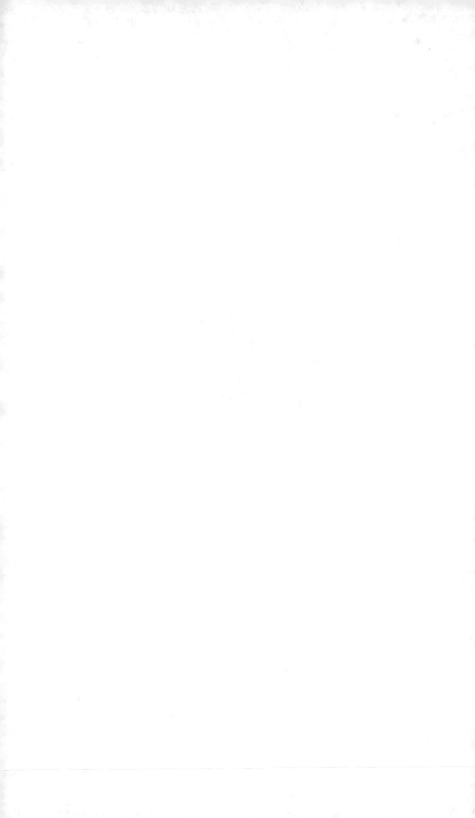

Printed in the United States
By Bookmasters